Pregnancy and Birth After Assisted Reproductive Technologies

Springer

Berlin
Heidelberg
New York
Barcelona
Hong Kong
London
Milan
Paris
Tokyo

Michael Ludwig

Pregnancy and Birth After Assisted Reproductive Technologies

Assisted by Constanze Banz, Georgine Huber,
Annika K. Schröder, Anna Sophie Seelig,
and Pia Wülfing

With a Foreword by Robert G. Edwards

With 3 Figures and 37 Tables

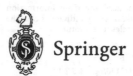 Springer

Author:

Priv.-Doz. Dr. Michael Ludwig
Department of Gynecology and Obstetrics, University Clinic
Div. of Reproductive Medicine and Gynecologic Endocrinology
Ratzeburger Allee 160, 23538 Lübeck, Germany

Contributors:

Dr. med. Constanze Banz   Dr. med. Georgine Huber
Dr. med Annika K. Schröder   Dr. med. Anna Sophie Seelig

Department of Gynecology and Obstetrics, University Clinic
Ratzeburger Allee 160, 23538 Lübeck, Germany

Dr. med. Pia Wülfing
Department of Gynecology and Obstetrics
Westfälische Universität Münster
Albert-Schweitzer-Strasse 33, 48149, Münster, Germany

ISBN 3-540-43531-X Springer-Verlag Berlin Heidelberg New York

Library of Congress Cataloging-in-Publication Data
Ludwig, Michael, 1968–. Pregnancy and birth after assisted reproductive
technologies / Michael Ludwig ; with contributions by Constanze Banz ... [et al.].
p. ; cm. Includes bibliographical references and index.
ISBN 354043531X (alk. paper)
1. Pregnancy – Complications. 2. Childbirth. 3. Human reproductive technology.
I. Title. [DNLM: 1. Pregnancy Complications. 2. Labor. 3. Reproductive Techniques,
Assisted – adverse effects. WQ 240 L948p 2002]   RG526 .L835 2002   618.3 – dc21
2002070466

Springer-Verlag Berlin Heidelberg New York
a member of BertelsmannSpringer Science+Business Media GmbH
http:/www.springer.de

© Springer-Verlag Berlin Heidelberg 2002
Printed in Germany

Cover design: E. Kirchner, Heidelberg
Typesetting: Fotosatz-Service Köhler GmbH, Würzburg

Printed on acid-free paper   SPIN 10875465   21/3130/op 5 4 3 2 1 0

**Dedicated to my teacher
Professor Dr. Klaus Diedrich**

Foreword

It is a pleasure to see this book in print. It represents work on an immense importance to assisted human conception. Numerous books have presented virtually every aspect of follicular growth, fertilization, male and female sterility and implantation. This is among the rare books dedicated to pregnancy, birth and infant growth.

Since the introduction of IVF, it has been clear that various problems could be associated with pregnancy after assisted human conception. The first clinical IVF pregnancy after the transfer of a 5-day blastocyst turned out to be ectopic, and this subject has never been far from debates on the safety of assisted human conception ever since. Ectopic and heterotopic pregnancies were two factors stressed in early days of worldwide IVF, and multiple pregnancies emerged as perhaps as an even more serious problem as high degrees of ovarian stimulation began to be practised in some clinics. These chapters add the experience of the author, working in a large German IVF team, to discussions on these topics in this book.

It is significant to note two chapters devoted to chromosomal analysis and preimplantation and prenatal diagnosis. A deeper awareness of the immense frequency of monosomic, trisomic and other chromosomally abnormal embryos must be stressed, since our species seems to be unique in this regard, and such pregnancies add to the stress of IVF. Today's methods promise to analyse these situations in immensely fine detail, almost to the molecular level, without chromosomes having to be analysed when in mitosis. New techniques constantly beckon, such as comparative genomic hybridization, to set the scene at ever-more detailed analyses of cleaving embryos, blastocysts and fetuses. Prenatal diagnosis is also essential, especially when more new methods involving non-invasive procedures are steadily introduced into IVF. This fallback form of diagnosis has been extremely significant since before the birth of Louise Brown, and is still immensely relevant today when new forms of ovarian stimulation, or ways of achieving conception, raise risks of more

and novel forms of chromosomal anomalies. Congenital malformations must also be closely monitored, especially since
recent reports indicate a slightly higher degree of them after
IVF and ICSI.

Perinatal outcome is the consequence of ovarian, embryonic and uterine aspects of conception. To record the frequency of congenital malformations at birth and one or two
years later is a very time-consuming and expensive task. Every
aspect of development could be influenced by disorders in
imprinting, uterine nutrition, and events at parturition in a
group of patients far beyond the mean ages of reproduction.
These effects could be transmitted to children and become
operative long after birth, as witnessed in reproductive
cloning in animal species. Even though a major task for any
author, Michael Ludwig has taken it in his stride to comple-
ment the earlier events determining child health at birth.

Chapters on oocyte donation, lesbian families, family
structure and gender identity complete the make-up of this
book. It could be a classic, consulted by clinical and scientific
investigators, and perhaps by patients and by general readers.
The author must have spent an immense amount of time
attending to fine detail in so many areas of pregnancy, parturition and early development. He is to be complimented
greatly on this vast effort.

August 2002   Robert G. Edwards

Preface

Assisted reproductive techniques have become more and more widespread throughout the world. It is estimated that about a million children have been born after an IVF procedure – taking all techniques together, the total must be much higher.

Together with the number of births, the number of studies investigating the course of the pregnancies and the health of the children has increased. Several predictions made even before the possibility of IVF became reality have not, however, come true.

Within this book we have striven to bring together as many publications as possible – including, hopefully, all of the most important studies to date – and to combine them into a coherent picture, not just single parts without a common thread. In doing this, we wanted to create a book which assists not only the specialist in reproductive medicine, but also the general obstetrician and everyone who has to counsel couples who undergo an ART treatment.

This book provides possible answers to a lot of questions that may arise in a dialogue with the infertile couple, based on established facts.

I would like to thank all my co-authors, who spent a great deal of time collecting and collating all the data from the different studies. I also thank Dr. Heilmann and Mrs. McHugh of Springer-Verlag for the opportunity to create this book and for their help with the final preparation of the manuscript.

We sincerely hope that this book proves as helpful as we intended.

Michael Ludwig

Contents

11 General Conclusions
Michael Ludwig 127

Abbreviation List 131

References 133

1 A Follow-up of Pregnancies in Assisted Reproduction: Necessity and Problems

Michael Ludwig

Different steps in any treatment of assisted reproductive technologies (ART) are important for the success of the treatment cycle. These are the means of ovarian stimulation, laboratory procedures, embryo transfer in in vitro fertilization (IVF) cycles, and luteal phase support. Throughout such a treatment cycle, the most important goal is to treat the woman as successfully as possible, but also to have as little impact as possible on the woman's health. However, the birth of a healthy child is the most important measure of quality control in any form of ART. On the other hand, this measure is also quite difficult to evaluate.

There seems to be no child born following an IVF procedure who has been subjected to more evaluation than Louise Brown, the result of the first successful IVF procedure in humans. The great interest in her development all through the years clearly shows that people do not really believe in the safety of such an unnatural means of reproduction as IVF.

In the past, different objections have been made towards IVF. It has been suggested that the "cold" conception might disturb the development of the child and the "warm" parent-child relationship. It has also been suggested that the involved doctor may act as a "third parent" and disturb the relationships between the parents and among the new developing IVF family.

The dangers of the IVF procedure – ethical and technical – were outlined well before the procedure was proven to be successful in humans. Most of these theoretical dangers have been chosen as topics of different studies, and, as shown by the different chapters in this book, most have proven not be to be realistic. Others, however, which could not be predicted, have been proven to have some basis in reality. We had also to learn that not everything we see in pregnancies and births after ART procedures can be explained by known factors – infertility per se seems to have a higher impact than previously believed.

The dilemma is that the course of a pregnancy, the birth and health of the child, and – even more importantly – the subsequent development of the child are difficult to assess. It is problematic that most IVF centres look very carefully to the quality of their treatment while the embryos are in the laboratory but are not able to extend this follow-up as far as the early pregnancy. During ovarian stimulation, induction of ovulation, collection of oocytes and transfer of embryos, the woman will be in very close contact with the IVF centre. Most centres also will see the patient up to the day of positive hCG at 14 to 16 days after embryo transfer. After that patients will normally go back to the referring physician who will take care of the pregnancy. Many centres will only become aware of spontaneous abortion, pregnancy termination or live birth following any complication of the pregnancy when the patient returns for a new treatment cycle. The follow-up procedure of other centres involves handing out postcards which have to be returned when the pregnancy comes to an end. Only a small number of centres are able to follow up their patients using standardized questionnaires at different time-points during the pregnancy as well as at the expected time of birth of the child.

Why Is It Necessary to Perform a Follow-up of Pregnancies After an ART Procedure?

The data in this book show that under certain circumstances problems will arise after an ART procedure with a higher frequency than after a spontaneous conception. For example, pregnancies resulting from conventional IVF will have a higher risk of premature birth and the newborn will more often be small for gestational age. Pregnancies established after intracytoplasmic sperm injection (ICSI) might have a higher risk of chromosomal, especially gonosomal, aberrations. A multiple birth is a well-known risk factor for the children, but may also lead to serious problems for the mother after the birth.

Patients who ask for an ART procedure are principally not interested in the rise in oestradiol levels, the quality of oocytes or their fertilization potential. They do not generally care about blastomere numbers or morphological criteria of embryo quality. However, they do finally come to realise that these factors might be important in predicting a clinical pregnancy because we tell them that they are. Principally, however, they are only interested in the baby take-home rate, and are particularly concerned as to whether their child will be in danger as a result of the chosen ART technique.

Even though oocyte pick-up, embryo transfer, a sufficient luteal phase, a positive hCG in serum and positive heart beats on ultrasound imaging might all be good end-points for clinical studies, they are not an end-point of treatment. Therefore, our counselling cannot concentrate on the dangers of infections from the use donor sperm, or of oocyte pick-up and ovarian hyperstimulation syndrome – it must extend to the risk of a multiple pregnancy or the risks that might be associated with the ART technique.

It may be reasonable to assume that patients know about the different risks, e.g. the risk of multiple pregnancies. Literature data, however, clearly show that despite sufficient counselling, patients do not. Gleicher et al. (1995) found that 65 % of 582 couples feared the problems of multiple pregnancies, and most were aware of the problems of even a twin pregnancy for the children and mother. On the other hand, 67 % of the patients explicitly wished to have twins. In contrast, Gleicher et al. found that 82 % of patients did not want to have a high-order multiple pregnancy, and 10 % would not accept twins (Gleicher et al. 1995). These data are confirmed by those of Goldfarb et al. (1996) (Tables 1.1, 1.2) indicating that, despite counselling and the fact that most couples are aware of the risks associated with multiple pregnancies, about two-thirds would be prepared to

Table 1.1. Results of a questionnaire on the estimation of risks of multiple pregnancies after special consultation (according to Goldfarb et al. 1996). *1* not tolerable at all, *2* more or less tolerable, *3* does not matter, *4* would be nice, *5* would be very nice

	Partner		Treatment	
	Female ($n = 77$)	Male ($n = 77$)	IVF ($n = 27$)	Intrauterine insemination ($n = 50$)
Singletons	4.9 ± 0.3	4.9 ± 0.2	4.9 ± 0.3	4.9 ± 0.2
Twins	4.7 ± 0.6	4.4 ± 1.0	4.5 ± 0.6	4.7 ± 0.5
Triplets	3.3 ± 1.1	3.1 ± 1.3	3.0 ± 1.4	3.4 ± 1.5
Quadruplets	2.2 ± 1.1	2.2 ± 1.1	2.0 ± 1.0	2.4 ± 1.1
More than quadruplets	1.8 ± 1.1	1.9 ± 1.0	1.5 ± 0.8	2.0 ± 1.2

Table 1.2. Results of a questionnaire. The question was whether couples would prefer not to be pregnant at all than face the possibility of triplets or quadruplets (data according to Goldfarb et al. 1996)

	Partner		Treatment	
	Female ($n = 77$)	Male ($n = 77$)	IVF ($n = 27$)	Intrauterine insemination ($n = 50$)
Triplets vs no pregnancy (%)	95	88	88	98
Quadruplets vs no pregnancy (%)	68	61	61	71

have twins. Therefore, counselling about the pregnancy, pregnancy course and birth by an IVF specialist is necessary.

But what should we counsel? Do we have an increased abortion rate following intrauterine insemination (IUI), IVF or ICSI? Do we have more chromosomal aberrations? Do we have to expect more complications during the pregnancy course or at birth? What about the health of the newborn, the possibility of a stillbirth? How does the child develop during the first years of life – do we have to expect abnormalities there? And, finally, how does the structure of the newly created family do? Is it comparable to a family where a pregnancy occurred spontaneously, perhaps incidentally, without any problems, without any hormones etc? How do the parents take care of the child; do they "overprotect" it? Do they expect too much from the so-much-wanted "idealized" child? There may be special situations in other circumstances. How do the parents deal with the fact of oocyte or sperm donation? Do they tell the child? If yes or no – how does the child react? What about single mothers or lesbian mothers? Does this harm the child's development?

Whatever those who are involved in reproductive medicine say about most of these questions, there is no doubt that, even though everything may proceed with no problem, we have to see the other side. We have to face the criticisms that nothing may go right, and that nothing is as it is under natural circumstances. We must also be aware that we do not live in a time in which it is sufficient to "believe" that everything is fine, to "suppose" that nothing will go wrong, or "to have the impression" or "gut feeling", that everything is as we say it is. When we counsel, we should counsel about things we can prove. And if we cannot prove them, because there are no reliable data, we must say so.

Why Do Not All Centres Perform a Follow-up of Pregnancies After an ART Procedure?

One has to be aware that the follow-up of an ART pregnancy is a quite difficult procedure – from the doctor's point of view and from the patient's point of view.

Some patients do not want to be confronted again and again with the problem of infertility. They just want to forget about the associated problems of infertility treatment, and go through the pregnancy as naturally as possible. This also leads to the fact that couples avoid speaking about the infertility treatment in the maternity hospital, or even avoid discussing it with the paediatrician who takes care of the child after birth and in the first years of life. This is, of course, their personal choice and must be accepted by everyone. On the other hand, it makes the complete, retrospective identification of these pregnancies and children nearly impossible.

From the doctor's point of view the follow-up of a pregnancy is also complicated. Even with a prospective approach, one has to expect to lose contact with about 2% of couples who move home and do not leave a new address. Retrospectively, this rate rises to about 15–20% after a 1–4 years (Ludwig et al. 1999a,b).

A sufficient follow-up should include several contacts with the pregnant couple:

- At 6–8 weeks of pregnancy to obtain information about a clinical vs a biochemical pregnancy.
- At 14–16 weeks of pregnancy to obtain information about clinical abortions, first sonographic evaluations such as nuchal translucency screening, or even pregnancy terminations following amniocentesis or chorionic villous sampling.
- At about 28–32 weeks of pregnancy to keep in contact with the couple and prospectively evaluate certain problems, premature labour, signs of preeclampsia and further sonographic evaluations such as fetal echocardiography or high-resolution ultrasound for the sonographic exclusion of malformations.
- At about 2 weeks after the expected date of birth to evaluate the final weeks of gestation, mode of delivery, complications at birth regarding mother and child, and to evaluate the health of the child, neonatal problems and malformations.

These contacts can be made either by post (low workload but high loss to follow-up) or by telephone (higher workload but lower loss to follow-up). Of course, a combined approach – first postal contact and then if no response a telephone contact – would be possible and might be reasonable as an optimal intermediate approach.

Assuming a centre will do about 1000 IVF cycles per year, with a pregnancy rate of 25 % and a delivery rate of 20 %, means that per year 250 pregnancies must be expected and 200 deliveries. Therefore, 850 telephone calls would be necessary to perform a close follow-up. Additionally time must be spent collecting the data in a computer system in a standardized manner. From our experience, each of these telephone contacts will take about 5 min, at least, resulting in an additional work load of 8 hours per month. It might be difficult to make telephone contact, bearing mind that several approaches may be necessary to contact the parents at different times in a day and that people may have to be contacted several times, since they may not reliably send data after only one phone call. It is therefore nearly impossible do this work and the computer documentation in addition to the routine work in most centres, and the additional costs incurred are not covered by the health insurance companies or the patients.

Additionally, even if different centres provide a follow-up of pregnancies and children born, this will not mean that all these data can be put together to generate a more reliable data set. Approaches might be different: some will perform a defined and prospective follow-up as outlined above, others will do a retrospective data collection. Other questions might arise: Have all centres included all abortions and induced abortions? What was the inclusion criterion for a "clinical" pregnancy: strongly rising hCG levels, a gestational sac on ultrasound, or positive fetal heart beats? What was the definition of early and late abortion, stillbirth, and live birth? Did all centres use a common definition of "major malformation"? What was the counselling with regard to prenatal invasive genetic diagnosis? What percentage of patients decided to have prenatal diagnosis?

To conclude, even if centres are willing to provide a close follow-up of their pregnancies and children, it would take a lot of standardization to compare these data between centres.

Conclusion

The discussion clearly shows that a follow-up is necessary for the process of counselling of couples who ask for infertility treatment. It also shows that these data are nearly impossible to collect during routine working time. Furthermore, data collection itself does not mean high quality, and certainly does not mean comparability.

Therefore, the most reliable data will not come from routine follow-up programs – if they exist at all – but from defined, large prospective studies. Data from registries might be helpful to identify time trends and to provide a rough idea about the techniques performed, frank risks, and distribution of treatments throughout a certain area, country or continent. They will, however, not provide a sufficient basis for a clear estimation of risks in the pregnancies and for the children born.

2 Incidence of Early Abortions and Ectopic Pregnancies in Assisted Reproduction

Annika K. Schröder, Michael Ludwig

Introduction

Spontaneous abortion is the most common complication of pregnancy. The incidence of spontaneous abortion after spontaneous conception is difficult to determine because most pregnancies are lost before clinical recognition (Wilcox et al. 1988). The incidence of spontaneous abortion after natural conception has been estimated to be between 10% and 15% of all clinically recognized pregnancies (Miller et al. 1980). Cytogenetic evaluations of these spontaneous abortions have shown that 50–70% of the embryos are chromosomally abnormal (Simpson 1980). The chromosomal abnormalities largely result from errors in meiotic division during gametogenesis and result in genetically abnormal embryos. Some authors have concluded that the incidence of clinical abortion is higher in pregnancies resulting from in vitro fertilization (IVF) or even from other forms of assisted reproduction than in those with natural conceptions (Rizk et al. 1991b). Such comparisons may be complicated by the use of different definitions of pregnancy and abortion, by different methods of calculating abortion rates, and by failing to take into account the gestational age at the time of abortion.

Definitions

IVF has required the coining of new categories of pregnancy outcome including preclinical and biochemical pregnancy, and its failure – e.g. preclinical abortion. It is difficult to compare abortion rates following IVF with those following natural conception, as the occurrence of pregnancies following natural conception is usually not established either as early or as precisely as after IVF and embryo transfer (ET). The cause of the infertility, maternal age and multiple gestation may also influence abortion rates.

Since the diagnosis of early pregnancy is complex and no standard definition exists, variations in estimated abortion rates in early pregnancy may simply reflect different definitions. This is especially true for biochemical pregnancies which are diagnosed solely on the basis of raised hCG values with no delay in menstrual period. A preclinical abortion has been defined by Jones et al. as a pregnancy diagnosed by two raised hCG values within 28 days of fertilization, i.e. when the menstrual period is delayed no more than 14 days (Jones et al.

1983). Such an abortion is usually indistinguishable from the normal menstrual period. A clinical abortion is defined as a spontaneous termination of pregnancy at least 28 days after fertilization but prior to viability, i.e. when the menstrual period is delayed by 14 days or more. Most authors mention the 16th week of gestation as an upper limit for an early clinical abortion, but not all authors who have reported an abortion rate in their study mention the upper limit of gestational age. This complicates the comparison of given numbers.

Incidence of Spontaneous Abortions

Since there might be a difference in the incidence of spontaneous abortions depending on the method used, the different techniques of assisted reproduction will be studied separately. Figure 2.1 gives an overview of all the techniques.

IVF

An analysis of the results from 75 individual groups is presented in "The World Collaborative Report on in Vitro Fertilisation and Embryo Replacement: Current State of the Art in January 1984" (Seppala 1985). ET was performed in 7993 cycles analysed. The overall pregnancy rate was 14.2%, and 285 (3.6%) biochemical pregnancies were detected. Abortion followed in 324 of 1084 clinically detected pregnancies (29.9%); 19 (1.8%) ectopic pregnancies were reported.

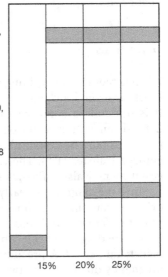

IVF: 15–30%
Seppala 1985, Wood 1985, Lindenberg 1985, Cohen 1986, Varma 1987, Saunders 1988, Sundstrom 1989, Roesler 1989, Sunde 1990, Mesrogli 1991, Wennerholm 1991, Shields 1992, Lancaster 1996, Govaerts 1998, Schmidt-Sarosi 1998, Strandell 1999, Van Golde 1999, AFS 1999, Westergaard 1999, AIDR 2000

ICSI: 15–25%
Wisanto 1995, Coulam 1996, Tarlatzis 1996, Govaerts 1998, Tarlatzis 1998, Van Golde 1999, Wennerholm 2000, Westergaard 2000, AIDR 2000

Donor insemination: 10–20%
David 1980, Katzorke 1981, Thepot 1996, Coulam 1996, Horne 1998

Cryotransfer: 20–30%
Van Steirteghem 1985, Coulam 1996, Al Hasani 1996, Simon 1998, Tarlatzis 1998

Spontaneous conception: 10–15%
Miller 1980

15%   20%   25%

Fig. 2.1. Incidence of abortions following different ART procedures

Wood and Trounson (1985) reported the outcome of 281 IVF pregnancies from 1980 to 1984. They report 65 (21.0%) biochemical pregnancies, 22 (7.1%) ectopic pregnancies and 79 (25.6%) spontaneous abortions. Varma et al. compared the outcome of infertility treatment in five different infertility groups (Varma and Patel 1987). Group 1 consisted of 181 patients treated with IVF for ovulatory dysfunction, group 2 consisted of 115 patients treated for male factor infertility including oligozoospermia, oligoasthenozoospermia and teratozoospermia, group 3 consisted of 72 patients undergoing insemination with donor spermatozoa because of azoospermia, group 4 consisted of 46 patients treated for tubal infertility and group 5 consisted of 86 patients who were investigated but conceived without treatment. Of the patients with tubal infertility (group 4), 40 underwent tubal surgery and 6 IVF treatment. The outcome in these patients was compared with the total obstetric population attending St. George's Hospital, London, who received similar management through pregnancy. The incidence of spontaneous abortion in patients with insemination with donor spermatozoa was significantly higher (13.8%) than the incidence in the other infertility groups and in the control group (6.2%; $P < 0.01$). The mean age of the women in group 3 who aborted was higher than the mean age of those with an ongoing pregnancy (35 years or older). The incidence of ectopic pregnancies was significantly higher in women with tubal infertility (21.7%) than in women in the other groups and the control group ($P < 0.01$). The results of a retrospective study by Varma and Patel (1987) and of another by Craft and Brinsden (1989) in which the clinical abortion rate in relation to the cause of infertility were analysed are summarized in Table 2.1. There is a notable difference in the abortion rates given in these studies, probably representing a difference in the quality of the studies.

Table 2.1. Two retrospective studies presenting the clinical abortion rate in relation to the cause of infertility

Study	Method	Cause of infertility	Clinical pregnancies n (%)[a]	Clinical abortions n (%)
Varma and Patel 1987	IVF	Ovulatory dysfunction	181	15 (8.3)
		Male infertility	115	9 (7.8)
		Azoospermia	72	10 (13.8)
		Tubal infertility	46	3 (6.5)
		No treatment	86	4 (4.7)
		No infertility	7893	491 (6.2)
Craft and Brinsden 1989	GIFT	Postinflammatory	56 (35.4)	19 (33.9)
		Endometriosis	22 (29.3)	4 (18.3)
		Idiopathic	116 (36.1)	28 (24.1)
		Ovulatory	7 (38.9)	2 (28.6)
		Polycystic ovary syndrome	18 (29.5)	7 (38.9)
		Male factor	141 (33.6)	35 (24.8)

[a] Percentages for clinical pregnancy rates were not available from the study of Varma and Patel (1987).

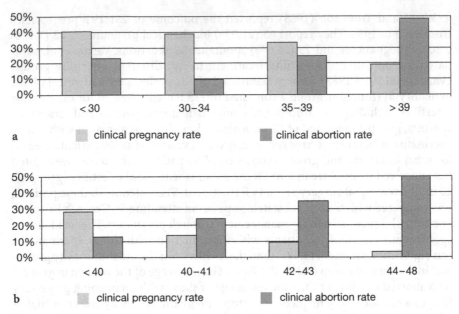

Fig. 2.2 a, b. Relationship between maternal age and pregnancy loss in (a) GIFT cycles (data according to Coulam et al. 1996) and (b) IVF cycles (data according to Lass et al. 1998)

The Australian IVF register noted 1192 pregnancies from 1979 to 1986. Of these pregnancies, 258 ended in a spontaneous abortion (22%), 62 in an ectopic pregnancy (5%), 33 (3%) in a stillbirth and 839 (70%) in a live birth (Saunders et al. 1988). The main cause of infertility in this cohort was tubal infertility (69%). Sundstrom and Wramsby in their IVF programme observed an early abortion rate (< 13 weeks of gestation) of 28% with an implantation rate of 9.2% and a pregnancy rate of 24.4% (Sundstrom and Wramsby 1989).

A retrospective analysis of all IVF cycles (6489 cycles) performed in Nordic countries from 1981 to 1987 showed a pregnancy rate of 13.3% with a spontaneous clinical abortion rate of 28.5% and 66 ectopic pregnancies (7.7%) (Sunde et al. 1990).

The United States 1989 In Vitro Fertilisation-Embryo Transfer (IVF-ET) Registry reported 3923 clinical pregnancies and 902 spontaneous abortions (23%) in patients undergoing either IVF or gamete intrafallopian transfer (GIFT) (SART 1992). The high rate of implantation failure in infertile couples after IVF is a major problem of this kind of treatment. Usually no information on the development of the embryo can be obtained during the time between ET and rising hCG levels.

Lass et al. (1998) have shown that with increasing maternal age the pregnancy rate decreases and the abortion rate increases. In patients under 40 years of age they observed an abortion rate of 12.7% after IVF, while in patients of 40–42 years of age they observed an abortion rate in the range of 21.7–28.2% (Fig. 2.2).

Table 2.2. Incidence of preclinical and clinical abortions after IVF (*n.a.* not available)

Study	Method	Embryo transfers (*n*)	Clinical pregnancies *n* (%)	Clinical abortions *n* (%)	Preclinical abortions *n* (%)
Seppala 1985	IVF	7,993	1084 (13.6)	324 (29.9)	285 (3.6)
Wood and Trounson 1985	IVF	n.a.	281	55	21 (7.5)
Lindenberg et al. 1985	IVF	25	3 (12.0)	3 (12.0)	n.a.
Cohen et al. 1986	IVF	n.a.	1163	n.a.	n.a.
Varma and Patel 1987	IVF	n.a.	414	37	n.a.
Saunders et al. 1988	IVF	n.a.	1192	258	n.a.
Sundstrom and Wramsby 1989	IVF	349	85 (24.4)	(28.0)	n.a.
Roesler et al. 1989	IVF	n.a.	130	26 (20.0)	n.a.
Sunde et al. 1990	IVF	6,489	852 (13.1)	242 (28.5)	n.a.
Mesrogli et al. 1991	IVF	82	12 (15.0)	3 (4.0)	2 (11.8)
Wennerholm et al. 1991	IVF	n.a.	206	(26.0)	n.a.
Shields et al. 1992	IVF, frozen ET, GIFT, ZIFT	720	213 (29.6)	65 (31.0)	n.a.
Lancaster 1996	IVF	n.a.	244	(27.0)	n.a.

Van Golde et al. analysed data from medical records of 120 pregnancies resulting from IVF and 113 pregnancies resulting from intracytoplasmic sperm injection (ICSI) (Van Golde et al. 1999). The pregnancy rate per transfer was 27 % for IVF and 23.2 % for ICSI. The rates of spontaneous abortions before 20 weeks of gestation were 22 of 120 (18.3 %) for IVF and 18 of 113 (15.9 %) for ICSI. The overall ongoing pregnancy rate after 20 weeks of gestation was 81.5 %. Therefore, there was no significant difference between ICSI and IVF in terms of outcome.

Data regarding abortion rates following conventional IVF are shown in Table 2.2.

GIFT

Craft and Brinsden analysed the data from 1071 cycles using GIFT. An overall pregnancy rate of 33.6% was achieved (Craft and Brinsden 1989). Age was a major factor influencing not only the pregnancy rate (40.2% in women < 30 years of age, 19.2% in women > 40 years of age, $P < 0.05$), but also the abortion rate which increased from 23.4% in women under 30 years of age to 48.4% in women over 40 years of age ($P < 0.05$). The lowest miscarriage rate was noted among women with endometriosis (18.2%), and the highest among women treated for polycystic ovary (PCO) syndrome (38.9%). Abortion rates in relation to causes of infertility are shown in Table 2.1.

Meirow and Schenker collected data relating to GIFT from world reports, national registries of different countries and meta-analysis of medical publications from 1986 to 1991. A total of 10,667 clinical pregnancies were reported with an abortion rate of 22.0% and an ectopic pregnancy rate of 5.5% (Meirow and Schenker 1995). Porcu et al. evaluated the outcome of transcervical GIFT with a falloscopic delivery system in 25 patients. The pregnancy rate was 28%, with no ectopic pregnancies observed. Spontaneous abortions occurred in 28.6% (Porcu et al. 1997).

ICSI

Because of the lack of natural selection of sperm with ICSI, concern about subsequent rates of pregnancy loss has been expressed. Govaerts et al. compared early pregnancy data in 50 ICSI pregnancies and 226 IVF pregnancies (Govaerts et al. 1996). They concluded that multiple pregnancies and miscarriage rates were not significantly different. The biochemical pregnancy rate was 16% in the ICSI and 17% in the IVF group. The miscarriage rate was 24% after ICSI and 29% after IVF. The incidence of vanishing twins was 16% of all twin pregnancies after ICSI and 25% after IVF. In 1998 the same group reported data on 145 pregnancies after ICSI that were matched with 145 pregnancies after IVF. The rates of preclinical (15% in ICSI and in IVF) and clinical abortions (11% in ICSI and 15% in IVF) were not different (Govaerts et al. 1998).

Coulam et al. compared the outcome of pregnancies after ICSI with those after IVF with fresh and frozen ET, and donor oocyte cycles (Coulam et al. 1996). A preclinical pregnancy loss was defined as one or more serum hCG concentrations of > 5 mIU/ml without a gestational sac seen by ultrasound. A clinical pregnancy loss was defined as a spontaneous or missed abortion occurring during the first trimester after visualizing a gestational sac by ultrasound. Of 136 pregnancies resulting from 405 ICSI cycles, 35 (26%) ended in preclinical loss and 28 (27.7%) ended in clinical loss, giving a total loss rate of 47%. After 201 cycles of conventional IVF, 71 pregnancies occurred, but 20 (28%) ended in a preclinical abortion and 13 (18%) in a clinical abortion. The preclinical and clinical abortion rates after donor oocyte cycles were 3% and 11%, respectively. When comparing pregnancies after oocyte donation cycles with pregnancies after IVF or ICSI in the homologous system, significantly fewer preclinical abortions occurred following oocyte donation compared with IVF ($P = 0.002$) or ICSI ($P = 0.003$).

When fresh ET after conventional IVF was compared with frozen ET, no significant difference in preclinical pregnancy losses was apparent ($P = 0.11$). No significant differences were observed in the frequencies of clinical pregnancy losses when pregnancies resulting from ICSI, IVF, donor oocyte cycles and frozen ET cycles were compared ($P = 0.2$). In addition, no differences were seen in the frequencies of chromosomal abnormalities in clinical pregnancy losses after various techniques of assisted reproduction. To determine whether preclinical or clinical pregnancy losses were related to semen quality, in the same study the frequency of pregnancy losses after ICSI was compared between four categories of semen (Coulam et al. 1996). Overall, no differences were observed among the various semen categories ($P = 0.33$). However, the authors could not exclude the possibility that differences between groups might appear with much larger sample sizes. The incidence of preclinical pregnancy loss increased with advancing female partner's age ($P = 0.01$), as did the rate of clinical pregnancy loss ($P = 0.02$). The outcome of pregnancy after frozen/thawed ET was similar to that after fresh ET.

Adonakis et al. analysed 525 ICSI cycles in 321 patients over the age of 40 years in order to determine whether the transfer of more than three embryos had a beneficial effect on the outcome of ICSI (Adonakis et al. 1997). The pregnancy rate was higher when at least four embryos were replaced. There were no statistically significant differences in the delivery rates or in the spontaneous abortion rate. When one to three embryos were transferred the abortion rate was 25.9% (pregnancy rate 11.8%) compared with 34.5% when four or more embryos were transferred (pregnancy rate 27.5%, $P > 0.0001$); this difference was not significant.

The European Society of Human Reproduction and Embryology (ESHRE) Task Force on ICSI is aiming to collect annually the clinical results and the pregnancy outcomes of ICSI on a worldwide basis using ejaculated, epididymal and testicular spermatozoa (Tarlatzis 1996; Tarlatzis and Bili 1998). During the 3 years 1993–1995 the number of participating centres performing ICSI rose from 35 to 101, and the total number of ICSI cycles performed in these centres increased from 3157 to 23,932 per year. In 1995 a fresh ET was performed in 15,407 ICSI cycles with ejaculated spermatozoa producing 5012 positive β-hCG tests (28.0%) which resulted in 464 (9.3%) preclinical abortions, 723 (14.4%) clinical abortions, 70 (1.4%) ectopic pregnancies and 3808 viable pregnancies (24.7% per cycle). In this register, clinical pregnancies which were terminated spontaneously before 20 weeks of gestation were considered to be clinical abortions. In ICSI cases with epididymal spermatozoa, a fresh ET was accomplished in 952 cases producing 311 positive β-hCG tests (29.8% per cycle) which resulted in 41 (12.7%) preclinical abortions, 34 (10.6%) clinical abortions, and 236 (21.8%) viable pregnancies. There were no ectopic pregnancies recorded. In ICSI cycles with testicular spermatozoa, 731 fresh ETs were performed producing 207 positive β-hCG tests (26.8%) which resulted in 20 (10.1%) preclinical

Table 2.3. Incidence of preclinical and clinical abortions after ICSI (*n.a.* not available)

Study	Method	Embryo transfers (*n*)	Clinical pregnancies *n* (%)	Clinical abortions *n* (%)	Preclinical abortions *n* (%)
Coulam et al. 1996	ICSI	405	101 (24.9)	28 (21.0)	35 (26.0)
Tarlatzis 1996	ICSI (ejaculated spermatozoa)	9,581	n.a.	454 (15.2)	311 (10.4)
	ICSI (epididymal spermatozoa)	373	n.a.	17 (13.3)	15 (11.7)
	ICSI (testicular spermatozoa)	161	n.a.	12 (20.0)	6 (10.0)
Wisanto et al. 1995	ICSI (ejaculated spermatozoa)	n.a.	785	(21.9)	n.a.
	ICSI (epididymal spermatozoa)	n.a.	37	(37.8)	n.a.
	ICSI (testicular spermatozoa)	n.a.	30	(33.3)	n.a.
Govaerts et al. 1998	ICSI	n.a.	145	11	15
Tarlatzis and Bili 1998	ICSI, fresh ET (ejaculated spermatozoa)	15,407	n.a.	723 (14.4)	464 (9.3)
	ICSI, fresh ET (epididymal spermatozoa)	952	n.a.	34 (10.6)	41 (12.7)
	ICSI, fresh ET (testicular spermatozoa)	731	n.a.	34 (15.6)	22 (10.1)
	ICSI, frozen ET (ejaculated spermatozoa)	3,146	n.a.	83 (15.8)	72 (13.7)
	ICSI, frozen ET (epididymal spermatozoa)	144	n.a.	2 (9.1)	3
	ICSI, frozen ET (testicular spermatozoa)	73	n.a.	34 (15.6)	22
Deutsches IVF Register 2000	ICSI	19,549	4825 (24.7)	1036 (21.5)	n.a.
Van Golde et al. 1999	ICSI	n.a.	113 (23.2)	18 (15.9)	n.a.
Wennerholm et al. 2000c	ICSI	n.a.	1293	(21.4)	n.a.
Westergaard et al. 2000	ICSI	n.a.	n.a.	(25.0)	n.a.

abortions, 34 (15.6%) clinical abortions, 1 (0.5%) ectopic pregnancy and 152 (18.7%) viable pregnancies. The ICSI results were similar during the 3-year period (1993–1995). The pregnancy outcome does not seem to be affected by the origin of the spermatozoa.

A Danish matched control study examining 5219 women demonstrated the highest rate of spontaneous abortions for ICSI pregnancies (25%) compared to IVF pregnancies (17%) (Westergaard et al. 2000). This difference between the two ART procedures was statistically significant ($P < 0.05$). No such differences were found in the rate of ectopic pregnancies between IVF and ICSI treatment (5.5% and 2.1%, respectively). The authors do not give an interpretation of the observations made.

An overview of the data regarding abortions after ICSI is given in Table 2.3.

Frozen/Thawed ET

After the transfer of frozen/thawed embryos derived from ICSI and IVF, Van Steirteghem et al. observed among 22 and 37 pregnancies a preclinical abortion rate of 40.9% for ICSI and 27.0% for IVF (no significant difference), respectively (Van Steirteghem et al. 1994).

The rate of pregnancy loss is similar between frozen/thawed ET cycles and fresh IVF/ET or ICSI cycles. Fasouliotis and Schenker reported a retrospective analysis of 381 frozen/thawed cycles during 1991–1993 and found a clinical pregnancy rate of 16.6% and a spontaneous abortion rate of 17.0% (Fasouliotis and Schenker 1996). Coulam et al. reported the frequency of pregnancy loss among 19 pregnancies following frozen/thawed ET (Coulam et al. 1996). After frozen ET, 11% of pregnancies ended in preclinical and 21% in clinical abortions. There were no significant differences in the clinical abortion rates between ICSI, IVF and frozen ET cycles. Al-Hasani et al. after 333 frozen/thawed ETs derived from IVF and 774 frozen/thawed ETs derived from ICSI observed 34 and 28 pregnancies (17% and 18%), respectively. Both groups showed a similar abortion rate of 20% (Al Hasani et al. 1996).

The ESHRE task force reported 3149 frozen/thawed ETs, of which 7–11% resulted in a viable pregnancy (Tarlatzis and Bili 1998). The use of frozen/thawed embryos from ejaculated spermatozoa resulted in 72 biochemical pregnancies (13.7%), 83 clinical abortions (15.8%) and 10 ectopic pregnancies (1.9), whereas the use of epididymal spermatozoa resulted in 3 biochemical pregnancies (13.6%), 2 clinical abortions (9.2%) and no ectopic pregnancies. In addition, the use of embryos from testicular spermatozoa resulted in 22 biochemical pregnancies (10.1%), 24 clinical abortions (15.6%) and 1 ectopic pregnancy (0.5%). The abortion rates did not differ from those after fresh ET.

Simon et al. (1998) compared the outcome of 83 and 204 transfer cycles of frozen/thawed embryos generated from conventional IVF and ICSI, respectively. Again, the abortion rate did not differ between the two groups (22.0% for IVF and 26.8% for ICSI).

The data from these studies are shown in Table 2.4.

Table 2.4. Incidence of preclinical and clinical abortions after the transfer of frozen/thawed embryos (*n.a.* not available)

Study	Method	Embryo transfers (*n*)	Clinical pregnancies *n* (%)	Clinical abortions *n* (%)	Preclinical abortions *n* (%)
Pergament et al. 1992	Frozen ET-IVF	n.a.	37	(27.0)	n.a.
	Frozen ET-ICSI	n.a.	33	(40.9)	n.a.
Coulam et al. 1996	Frozen ET	87	19 (22.0)	4 (21.9)	2 (11.0)
Coulam et al. 1996	Frozen ET	n.a.	(16.6)	(17.0)	n.a.
Al Hasani et al. 1996	Frozen ET-IVF	n.a.	34	(20.0)	n.a.
	Frozen ET-ICSI	n.a.	28	(20.0)	n.a.
Simon et al. 1998	Frozen ET-IVF	83	n.a.	(22.0)	n.a.
	Frozen ET-ICSI	204	n.a.	(26.8)	n.a.
Tarlatzis and Bili 1998	Frozen ET-ICSI (ejaculated spermatozoa)	3146	n.a.	83 (15.8)	72 (13.7)
	Frozen ET-ICSI (epididymal spermatozoa)	144	n.a.	2 (9.1)	3
	Frozen ET-ICSI (testicular spermatozoa)	73	n.a.	34 (15.6)	22
Tarlatzis and Bili 1998	Frozen ET	2755	367 (13.3)	82 (22.3)	n.a.

Artificial Insemination with Donor Sperm (AID)

In a cohort of 1188 women who underwent AID using frozen sperm, David et al. observed a spontaneous abortion rate of 17% (David et al. 1980). A similar abortion rate of 18.4% was reported in a survey of 103 conceptions after AID (Chong and Taymor 1975). Katzorke et al. evaluated the outcome of 415 women treated with AID which resulted in 210 pregnancies after an average of 7.1 insemination cycles (Katzorke et al. 1981). The abortion rate was 15%, comparable to that in the fertile population. In another study of 168 pregnancies achieved by AID, the abortion rate was 12.5% (Lansac et al. 1983). Virro and Shewchuk reviewed the pregnancy outcome of 242 conceptions after AID. The spontaneous abortion rate was 17.4%. The incidence of spontaneous abortion was related to the number of cycles required per conception (Virro and Shewchuk 1984). A further study of 1345 pregnancies resulting from AID showed an 18% incidence of abortion (Schwartz et al. 1986). The abortion rate did not depend on any of the basic semen characteristics including the post-thaw motility, the factor most strongly linked to conception rate.

Table 2.5. Incidence of preclinical and clinical abortions after assisted insemination with donor sperm (AID) (*n.a.* not available)

Study	Method	Embryo transfers (*n*)	Clinical pregnancies *n* (%)	Clinical abortions *n* (%)	Preclinical abortions *n* (%)
Thepot et al. 1996	AID	n.a.	11,535	(17.7)	n.a.
Horne et al. 1998	AID	1465	248 (16.9)	39 (15.7)	n.a.
Coulam et al. 1996	AID	69	35 (51.0)	4 (11.0)	1 (3.0)
David et al. 1980	AID	n.a.	n.a.	(17.0)	n.a.
Katzorke et al. 1981	AID	n.a.	210	(15.0)	n.a.
Chong and Taymor 1975	AID	n.a.	103	(18.4)	n.a.

In their study mentioned above, Varma et al. included one group of 72 patients whose husbands were azoospermic and needed AID (Varma and Patel 1987). Among these 72 pregnancies there were 10 abortions (13.9%) and 2 ectopic pregnancies (2.7%). Amuzu et al. (1990) evaluated 594 pregnancies of women who conceived by AID. The spontaneous abortion rate was 16.5%, with no difference between fresh and frozen semen samples. However, significant correlations were found between abortion rate and maternal age ($P < 0.001$) and abortion rate and cycle of conception ($P < 0.025$), confirming the findings of others (Virro and Shewchuk 1984). Thepot et al. reported a spontaneous abortion rate of 17.7% in their series of 11,535 pregnancies with a known outcome after AID and an ectopic pregnancy rate of 0.8% (Thepot et al. 1996).

In a retrospective study of AID (Horne et al. 1998), 389 patients were found to have undergone 1465 procedures. The clinical pregnancy rate per cycle was 16.9% (248/1465). The rate of pregnancy loss was 15.7% (39/248) with a viable pregnancy rate of 14.3% (209/1465).

All studies regarding abortions following AID are shown in Table 2.5.

Incidence of Ectopic Pregnancies

The first pregnancy achieved using the IVF technique resulted in an ectopic pregnancy (Steptoe and Edwards 1976). Women who become pregnant by assisted conception would be expected to be at an increased risk of ectopic pregnancy because of the higher prevalence of tubal damage. Thus it is not surprising that ectopic pregnancies occur more often in IVF pregnancies compared with 1% after natural conception (Table 2.6).

In "The World Collaborative Report on in Vitro Fertilisation and Embryo Replacement: Current State of the Art in January 1984" the rate of ectopic pregnancies was reported as 1.8% (19 of 1084 pregnancies) (Seppala 1985). Wood and Trounson reported a similar rate of 2.1% in their series of IVF patients (Wood and Trounson 1985). The Australian IVF register recorded 62 ectopic pregnancies (5%) among 1192 pregnancies from 1979 to 1986. The main cause

Table 2.6. Ectopic pregnancies (*n.a.* not available)

Study	Design	Method	Pregnancies	
			Total	Extrauterine *n* (%)
Seppala 1985	Retrospective	IVF	1084	19 (1.8)
Wood and Trounson 1985	Retrospective	IVF	281	6 (2.1)
Cohen et al. 1986	Retrospective	IVF	1163	(5.0)
Saunders et al. 1988	Retrospective	IVF	1192	62 (5.0)
Craft and Brinsden 1989	Retrospective	GIFT	1071	25 (6.9)
Sunde et al. 1990	Retrospective	IVF	852	66 (7.7)
Wennerholm et al. 1991	Retrospective	IVF	206	
Thepot et al. 1996	Retrospective	IUI-donor	11535	92 (0.8)
Tarlatzis 1996	Retrospective	ICSI (ejaculated spermatozoa)	2595	51 (1.7)
		ICSI (epididymal spermatozoa)	110	2 (1.6)
		ICSI (testicular spermatozoa)	52	1 (1.7)
Tarlatzis and Bili 1998	Retrospective	ICSI, fresh ET (ejaculated spermatozoa)	4531	70 (1.4)
		ICSI, fresh ET (epididymal spermatozoa)	270	0 (0)
		ICSI, fresh ET (testicular spermatozoa)	186	1 (0.5)
		ICSI, frozen ET (ejaculated spermatozoa)	424	10 (1.9)
		ICSI, frozen ET (epididymal spermatozoa)	15	0 (0)
		ICSI, frozen ET (testicular spermatozoa)	39	1 (0.5)
Deutsches IVF Register 2000	Prospective	IVF	4400	144 (3.3)
		ICSI	4825	105 (2.2)
		Frozen ET	367	28 (7.6)
Strandell et al. 1999a	Retrospective	IVF	725	(4.0)
Van Golde et al. 1999	Retrospective	IVF	120	3 (2.5)
Wennerholm et al. 2000c	Retrospective	ICSI	1293	(1.2)
Westergaard et al. 2000	Retrospective	IVF	5219	(2.1)
	Retrospective	ICSI	n.a.	(5.5)

of infertility in this series was tubal infertility (69%). Serour et al. noted an ectopic pregnancy rate in their cohort of 1.9% among a total of 702 pregnancies (Serour et al. 1998). Marcus and Brinsden observed 135 ectopic pregnancies (4.5%) among 3000 clinical pregnancies after IVF (Marcus and Brinsden 1995). Of these ectopic pregnancies 20 were heterotopic (6.7‰). The main risk factor identified was a history of pelvic inflammatory disease ($P < 0.001$). There was slight evidence with marginal significance ($P = 0.05$) that patients having ectopic pregnancies received a higher volume of culture medium than those having normal deliveries. There was also a trend ($P = 0.07$) towards an association between high progesterone/oestradiol ratio on the day of ET and ectopic pregnancy. There was no statistically significant evidence of an association between ectopic pregnancy and a history of ectopic pregnancy, abortion, stillbirth, termination of pregnancy, neonatal death, tubal surgery, ovarian stimulation protocol, number of oocytes retrieved, number or quality of embryos transferred or the number of patent fallopian tubes.

Varma and Patel (1987) analysed the incidence of ectopic pregnancies after IVF in relation to the cause of the infertility. Ectopic pregnancies were observed in 21.7% of patients with tubal damage, but only in 0.5%–2.7% of patients with other causes of infertility and normal fallopian tubes ($P < 0.01$). It is interesting to note that the ectopic pregnancy rate observed after ICSI is 0–1.4% and appears to be considerably lower than the 4.3% reported after conventional IVF (de Mouzon and Lancaster 1993).

Craft et al. analysed the data from 1071 cycles using GIFT (Craft and Brinsden 1989). The rate of ectopic pregnancy was 6.9%. The highest rate occurred in women in whom the predominant factor of their infertility was postinflammatory sequelae or endometriosis (14.3% and 13.6%, respectively). The lowest rate occurred in women with idiopathic or male factor infertility (4.3% and 5.0%, respectively). Sunde et al. even reported a rate of ectopic pregnancy of 7.7% following IVF. In the their cohort, 82.6% of all patients were treated for impaired tubal function (Sunde et al. 1990).

Marcus et al. compared the data from 135 patients with an ectopic pregnancy with the data from 135 patients with a singleton delivery after IVF (Marcus et al. 1995). The mean plasma concentrations of hCG and progesterone were significantly lower in the ectopic pregnancy group compared to the singleton delivery group ($P < 0.001$). However, there was such a degree of overlap that it was impossible to devise a cut-off concentration for either hormone which would offer a clinically useful predictor of ectopic pregnancy.

Thepot et al. noted an ectopic pregnancy rate of 0.8% after intrauterine insemination with donor spermatozoa, reflecting the low rate of tubal damage in such a cohort of patients (Thepot et al. 1996). A retrospective analysis by Van Golde et al. (1999) revealed 3 ectopic pregnancies among 120 IVF pregnancies (2.5%), while there were no ectopic pregnancies following ICSI. Strandell et al. (1999a) studied a total of 725 women who conceived after IVF. The rate of ectopic pregnancies was 4%, corresponding to 29 ectopic pregnancies of which 2 were heterotopic (2.8‰). Tubal factor infertility, various previous abdominal surgeries, previous ectopic pregnancies or pelvic infection, presence of hydrosalpinx or fibroid, and the type of transfer catheter used showed a positive correlation with the occurrence of ectopic pregnancy. Logistic regression analysis, however, identified only two factors with predictive power: tubal factor infertility and previous myomectomy.

In a Danish matched control study examining 5219 women, no statistically significant difference was found in rates of ectopic pregnancy following IVF and ICSI treatment, which were 5.5% and 2.1%, respectively (Westergaard et al. 2000). However, the number of ectopic pregnancies was twofold higher in the IVF group. In a cohort of 234 pregnancies after IVF or IVF plus ICSI, eight ectopic pregnancies were observed, resulting in an ectopic pregnancy rate of 3.4% (Ludwig et al. 2001a).

Confirming the collected experience discussed above, ectopic pregnancies were shown to occur less often after the use of fresh or frozen/thawed embryos derived from ICSI (0–1.9%) (Tarlatzis and Bili 1998) than after IVF (Tarlatzis 1996). As ICSI is predominantly used for the treatment of male factor infertility the prevalence of tubal damage is lower in couples undergoing ICSI. Therefore, ectopic pregnancies are observed less frequently in this group of patients.

Incidence of Heterotopic Pregnancies

Heterotopic pregnancy is estimated to occur in 1% of pregnancies following IVF compared to 0.003% of spontaneous pregnancies. There are numerous case reports of heterotopic pregnancies after ART. Raziel et al. even reported the case of a recurrent heterotopic pregnancy in the same patient after IVF/ICSI in a 1 year period (Raziel et al. 1997). The first ended in emergency salpingectomy and missed intrauterine abortion. The second was managed by laparoscopic salpingectomy, and the synchronous intrauterine pregnancies ended in the delivery of twins. However, only large cohorts have sufficient power to estimate the real incidence of heterotopic pregnancies.

In 1991 Rizk et al. reported 17 cases of heterotopic pregnancies among 1648 clinical pregnancies (1.0%) (Rizk et al. 1991c). In a Danish survey the frequency of heterotopic pregnancies was 1.1% (13/1171) (Svare et al. 1993). In a study by Tummon et al. of 587 IVF pregnancies, 7 heterotopic pregnancies and 24 solely ectopic pregnancies were identified, all in the subset of 328 women (Tummon et al. 1994). Therefore, heterotopic pregnancies occurred in 2% of gestations after IVF, all in women with distorted tubal anatomy. Symptoms, signs and time of diagnosis were not different between heterotopic and solely ectopic pregnancies.

Compared with solely ectopic pregnancies, heterotopic pregnancies were associated with transfer of more embryos. With four or more embryos transferred the odds ratio for the development of heterotopic versus solely ectopic gestation was 10.0. In the cohort of Marcus and Brinsden, 135 ectopic pregnancies (4.5%) including 20 heterotopic pregnancies (0.67%) were observed in 3000 pregnancies after IVF. In another study, an ectopic pregnancy rate of 7.5% with a heterotopic pregnancy rate of 1.5% was found among all IVF pregnancies (2356 cycles, pregnancy rate per transfer 24%) (Mantzavinos et al. 1996). Three out of seven ectopic pregnancies (43%) were successfully continued with normal intrauterine embryo development and delivery. Serour et al. found a heterotopic pregnancy rate of 0.2% in a total of 702 pregnancies following IVF with an ectopic pregnancy rate of 1.9% (Serour et al. 1998). Hulvert et al. found 23 ectopic pregnancies (3.7%) in 618 pregnancies after an ART procedure. Seven of the 23 ectopic pregnancies were heterotopic (1.14%) (Hulvert et al. 1999). In the study mentioned above, Strandell et al. noted 29 ectopic pregnancies in 725 pregnancies of which 2 were heterotopic (0.27%) (Strandell et al. 1999a).

As a result of the widespread use of ART, heterotopic pregnancies are no longer a rarity. One has to be aware that the existence of an intrauterine gestation does not preclude the risk of nidation of other embryos in ectopic sites. Heterotopic pregnancies are more than 300 times more frequent after an ART procedure compared to spontaneous conception cycles.

Incidence of Disappearing Gestational Sacs

Disappearing gestational sacs seen on ultrasound during early pregnancy are no longer visible as the pregnancy progresses. Tan and Riddle scanned 140 intrauterine pregnancies after IVF from the 5th to the 13th week of pregnancy and the number of gestational sacs seen on ultrasound was recorded (Tan et al. 1989). In patients with one gestational sac seen on ultrasound, 27% of these sacs disappeared, in patients with two sacs 25% disappeared, and in those with three sacs 47% disappeared. The percentage of women who ended up without a viable pregnancy was 28%, 6% and 0%, respectively, for those who initially started with one, two and three sacs.

Is There a Higher Abortion Risk Following ART?

Data from different studies worldwide show quite varying degrees of abortion rates. However, the data seem to show that abortion rates are higher following conventional IVF than following other techniques of assisted reproduction (ICSI, donor insemination). Following cryopreservation, the rates are in a similar range (Fig. 2.1). On the other hand, however, there are also studies showing higher pregnancy loss rates for ICSI than for IVF. Therefore, this discussion is still ongoing.

It is difficult to provide a definitive argument as to why abortion rates are always higher following assisted reproduction than following natural conception. Different biases have to be taken into account. First, more pregnancies might be detected at an earlier time-point than following natural conception. These pregnancies, which normally would end as a preclinical abortion might be prolonged by hormonal supplementation using gestagens or additionally oestrogens. This leads to detection of these pregnancies at a clinical level, at the latest when a D&C is performed because of missed abortion and a highly proliferated endometrium. The higher rate of abortion in the IVF population might be explained by a higher rate of endocrinologically abnormal patients as compared to the other studied groups.

Since the introduction of ICSI as the treatment of choice for severe male factor infertility, caution about pregnancy outcome has been voiced because of the lack of natural selection of sperm. So far the studies that have compared IVF and ICSI have shown no differences in the pregnancy rate or the abortion rate between the two techniques.

The rate of preclinical or clinical pregnancy abortion has been shown to increase with advancing oocyte donor age. The association of advanced maternal age and the risk of spontaneous abortion is well known and has been shown to be related to the increased risk of embryonic chromosomal abnormalities with advanced maternal age (Munne et al. 1993, 1995) (Table 2.7). Munne et al. analysed 524 cleavage-stage human embryos obtained by IVF by fluorescence in situ hybridization (Munne et al. 1995). As shown in Table 2.7, the embryos were allocated into three groups according to morphological and developmental characteristics. The embryos were also analysed according to maternal age. It was demonstrated that in morphologically and developmentally normal human embryos, cleavage-stage aneuploidy significantly increases with maternal age. The lower preclinical pregnancy losses among recipients of fresh embryos from donor oocyte cycles could be due to better quality of embryos resulting from oocytes from younger women.

It is difficult to compare abortion rates following assisted reproduction with the rate following natural conception, as the occurrence of pregnancies following natural conception is usually not established either as early or as precisely as after any ART procedure. Therefore, more pregnancy losses are detected in women undergoing infertility treatment.

An increase in abortion rate after assisted reproduction compared to natural conception might be a result of the increased age of couples undergoing infertility treatment. The implantation rate as well as the miscarriage rate is significantly affected by the woman's age and therefore primarily by oocyte and

Table 2.7. Comparison of chromosome abnormalities in arrested, slow and/or fragmented and good embryos by maternal age (data from Munne et al. 1995)

	Maternal age group (years)		
	20–34	35–39	40–47
Total aneuploidy (%)			
Arrested embryos	5.5	5.6	10.4
Slow embryos	6.0	15.6	29.5
Good embryos	4.0	9.4	37.2
Total polyploidy (%)			
Arrested embryos	45.5	40.5	49.1
Slow embryos	8.7	15.5	13.5
Good embryos	4.0	2.1	1.1

IVF: 2–8%
Seppala 1985, Wood 1985, Cohen 1986, Saunders 1988, Craft 1998,
Sunde 1990, Wennerholm 1991, Van Golde 1999, Strandell 1999,
Westergaard 2000, AIDR 2000

ICSI: 1–2%
Tarlatzis 1996, Tarlatzis 1998, Deutsches IVF-Register 2000,
Wennerholm 2000, Westergaard 2000

Donor insemination: 1%
Thepot 1996

Spontaneous conception: 1%

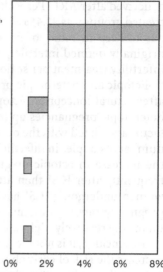

0%   2%   4%   6%   8%

Fig. 2.3. Graphic to show the estimation of ectopic pregnancies after different ART procedures

embryo quality (Tarlatzis and Bili 2000). Early abortions happen more frequently in women treated for PCO syndrome compared to other causes of infertility. A lot of women with PCO syndrome do not conceive spontaneously and have to undergo infertility treatment. Therefore, although the percentage of patients with PCO syndrome is rather small in relation to all patients undergoing IVF, the abortion rate of these women may influence the overall abortion rate in assisted reproduction.

Recent research has also shown that there might be an influence of maternal weight independent of the presence of an associated PCO. In one retrospective data analysis, a maternal body mass index of ≥ 25 kg/m^2 was found to be associated with a 1.77-fold increased risk (95% CI 1.05–2.97) of an early abortion, i.e. an abortion before 6 weeks of gestation after diagnosis by an increased hCG (i.e. a value above 10 IU/l) (Fedorcsak et al. 2000).

The number of embryos transferred does not seem to influence the abortion rate. There seems to be no difference in the frequency of abortions when comparing different techniques of assisted reproduction. In addition to this, the abortion rates following fresh and frozen/thawed cycles do not differ. Using ICSI it has been shown that the quality of sperm does not influence the frequency of abortions.

To really answer the question as to whether there is or there is not an increased risk of abortion following ART, a prospective controlled study is necessary in which pregnancies after natural conception starting about 14 days after conception would also be followed up. These data are, to the best of our knowledge, not yet available. There is one retrospective study on those patients, who either conceived spontaneously before infertility treatment was started, or conceived after ART (Pezeshki et al. 2000). The spontaneous abortion rate in the treated groups was 22.4% as compared to 26.2% in the non-treated patients. One has to keep in mind, of course, that the non-treated group also consisted of originally defined infertile patients. However, the study clearly shows that the infertility treatment per se does not increase the risk of spontaneous abortion.

Ectopic and heterotopic pregnancies are observed more often after IVF than after natural conception: ectopic pregnancies up to four to five times more often, heterotopic pregnancies up to 300 times more often. Tubal damage is the main factor associated with the occurrence of ectopic pregnancies (Fig. 2.3). The high number of couples in infertility programmes treated for tubal infertility explains the increase in ectopic pregnancies after IVF. Ectopic pregnancies occur less frequently after ICSI than after IVF. This difference is probably because most women undergoing ICSI have normal fallopian tubes. The increased multiple pregnancy rate in combination with the increased ectopic pregnancy rate explains the relatively high rate of heterotopic pregnancies.

To conclude, it is not the techniques that are used for infertility treatment that increase the risk of early abortion, and ectopic and heterotopic pregnancies, but the way these kinds of early pregnancy complications and risk factors associated with the infertility per se are recorded. Only heterotopic pregnancies seem to be associated with one aspect of ART techniques – the transfer of several embryos instead of one.

3 Incidence of Chromosomal Abnormalities in Abortions After Assisted Reproduction

Annika K. Schröder, Michael Ludwig

The contribution of chromosomal disorders to embryonic and fetal loss is well documented in humans. A 0.6% incidence of chromosomal abnormalities has been reported for live births (Nielsen 1975), a 10-fold increase in stillborns (6%) (Machin and Crolla 1974) and a 100-fold increase in spontaneous abortions (60%) (Boue and Boue 1976). It can be calculated that non-disjunction occurring in oocytes (11–65%) (Spielmann et al. 1985; Plachot et al. 1986, 1987b) or in fertilizing spermatozoa (8%) (Martin 1984) accounts for the high rate of chromosomal disorders in preimplantation embryos (29.6–71.7%) (Plachot et al. 1987a; Wimmers and van der Merwe 1988).

The developmental capacities of chromosomally abnormal embryos during the first 5 days in vitro depend on the degree of ploidy. The earliest lethal abnormality is a tetraploidy leading to a cleavage arrest at about eight cells. Some of the haploid embryos and the majority of triploid embryos reach the morula stage, and a few are even capable of developing into an early blastocyst (Plachot

Table 3.1. Incidence of chromosomal abnormalities in abortuses in assisted reproduction

Study	Method	Number of abortuses	Chromosome anomalies, n (%)
Boue and Boue 1976	In vivo		1498 (61.5)
Plachot 1989		34	21 (61.8)
Coulam et al. 1996	ICSI	15	11 (73.0)
	IVF	8	6 (75.09
	Oocyte donation	3	1 (33.3)
	Frozen ET	2	1 (50.0)
Schmidt-Sarosi et al. 1998	IVF, insemination	52	36 (69.2)
Shields et al. 1992	Frozen ET, IVF, GIFT, ZIFT	18	9 (50.0)
Lindenberg et al. 1985	IVF	3	1
Stern et al. 1996	IVF	224	128
Barlow et al. 1988	IVF	8	3
Roesler et al. 1989	IVF	13	6
le Porrier et al. 1988	IVF	13	7

Table 3.2. Chromosomal analysis of abortuses (*m* mosaic)

	Boue and Boue 1976	Barlow et al. 1988	Roesler et al. 1989	Plachot 1989	Shields et al. 1992	Stern et al. 1996	Schmidt-Sarosi et al. 1998
Method	In vivo	IVF	IVF	IVF	fPN, IVF, GIFT, ZIFT	IVF	IVF, insemination
Total number of abortuses	2	5	21	9	128	36	
Monosomy, *n* (%)	(15.3)	0	0	3 (14.2)	1 (1 m) (11.1)	6 (4.6)	2 (5.5)
Trisomy, *n* (%)	(52.0)	1 (1 m) (50.0)	4 (80.0)	14 (1 m) (61.9)	5 (1 m) (55.6)	100 (78.1)	24 (66.6)
Double trisomy, *n* (%)	(1.7)	1 (50.0)	0	1 (4.8)	0	0	2 (5.5)
Triploidy, *n* (%)	(19.9)	0	0	1 (4.8)	0	15 (11.7)	3 (8.3)
Tetraploidy, *n* (%)	(6.2)	0	1 (1 m) (20.0)	1 (4.8)	2 (1 m) (22.2)	7 (5.5)	0
Translocation, *n* (%)	(3.8)	0	0 (0)	1 (4.8)	0	0	1 (2.7)
Inversion, *n* (%)	0	0	1 (20.0)	0	1 (1 m) (11.1)	0	0
Mosaicism, *n* (%)	0	1 (50.0)	1 (20.0)	1 (4.8)	4 (44.4)	0	0

et al. 1988a). The ongoing debate as to whether there might be an increased risk of abortions following IVF has led to the theory that there might be an increased risk of chromosomal abnormalities in those embryos. The limited data on patients undergoing assisted reproduction that are available are shown in Tables 3.1 and 3.2 which show the incidence of chromosomal abnormalities and chromosomal analyses, respectively.

Monosomy

Monosomy X is one of the most common anomalies in spontaneous abortions. Incidences of 14.2% in the study by Plachot (1989) and 11.1% in the study by Shields et al. (1992) are close to the incidence reported after in vivo fertilization (15.3%) (Boue et al. 1975; Boue and Boue 1976). Autosomal monosomies should occur with the same frequencies as trisomies. Yet they are observed only exceptionally (in 0.1%) after in vivo fertilization, and are therefore considered to be responsible for preclinical abortions (Boue et al. 1975; Boue and Boue 1976). It has been reported that in the mouse preimplantation development and survival of monosomic embryos depend on a missing chromosome. Monosomy for autosomes 1, 3, 6, 16 and 19 does not affect cleavage, compaction and blastulation, and in some cases it is compatible with implantation. The cleavage of most of these embryos, however, stops as early blastocysts (monosomies 3, 16, 19) and some of them are eliminated during early postimplantation stages (monosomies 1 and 16) (Baranov 1983). Stern et al. have observed embryonic monosomy in only 6 of 224 cases of spontaneous abortion after IVF (4.8% of chromosomal abnormalities) (Stern et al. 1996). Schmidt-Sarosi et al. report a similar rate of 5.5% (Schmidt-Sarosi et al. 1998).

Trisomy

Trisomies for A, D, E and G chromosome groups represent 66.6% of all anomalies in aborted embryos. In contrast to the monosomies in which the missing chromosome is almost always a sex chromosome, in trisomies the extra chromosome is nearly always an autosome. In abortions, trisomies for all groups of chromosomes are found, but their relative frequencies are different. Trisomies C, D, E and G are frequent, whereas trisomies A, B and F are rare. A double trisomy has been observed by Plachot (1989). This double non-disjunction occurring in only 1.7% of abortuses after in vivo fertilization is frequently encountered in human oocytes: 15% are hyperhaploid, 10% show two extra chromosomes (Plachot et al. 1988b). The resulting embryos with several extra-autosomal chromosomes probably stop development before or just after implantation, as they are never encountered in first-trimester abortions.

The rate of trisomies in chromosomally abnormal abortuses after assisted reproduction varies between 50% (Barlow et al. 1988) and 80% (Roesler et al. 1989). Plachot reported an incidence of 61.9% (Plachot 1989) and Schmidt-Sarosi et al. 66.6% (Schmidt-Sarosi et al. 1998). Shields et al. observed autosomal trisomies in 55.6% of abortuses (Shields et al. 1992). Stern et al. reported fetal trisomy in 100 of 224 cases (44.6%) of spontaneous abortions, and 128 of these abortuses showed chromosomal abnormalities. Therefore fetal trisomy accounts for 78.1% of chromosomal abnormalities (Stern et al. 1996). The variations of the given incidences might be a result of the small numbers of cases in each series.

Advanced maternal age is known to be associated with meiotic non-disjunction leading to trisomic conceptions. The frequency of these abnormalities is higher in early pregnancies when genetic evaluation, i.e. chorionic villous sampling or amniocentesis is performed, than at birth due to spontaneous loss of aneuploid conceptions. The mean maternal age in the study by Shields et al. was 36.3 years (Shields et al. 1992). The incidence of trisomy in the chromosomally abnormal cases (55.6%) was similar to that reported by Boue et al. (1975) in abortuses of less than 12 weeks gestation (52%) (Boue and Boue 1976). Boue et al. gave an average maternal age of 31.3 years for conceptions with trisomies (Boue and Boue 1976), while the series of Shield et al. had an average maternal age of 34.4 years for these conceptions (Shields et al. 1992).

Triploidy

Triploidy accounts for 19.9% of all anomalies found in spontaneous abortions after in vivo fertilization (Boue et al. 1975; Boue and Boue 1976). Plachot et al. observed one case of triploidy in their survey (4.8%) (Plachot 1989). Stern et al. noted a fetal triploidy in 11.7% (15/128) of chromosomally abnormal fetuses (Stern et al. 1996), and Schmidt-Sarosi et al. in 8.3% of chromosomally abnormal fetuses (Schmidt-Sarosi et al. 1998). According to Plachot the incidence at conception is higher after in vitro (about 6%) than after in vivo fertilization (about 1.5%) because of the high number of inseminated spermatozoa after IVF and the risk of oocyte ageing. The possibility of detecting triploid eggs the day after insemination might decrease the incidence at implantation after IVF (Plachot 1989). Using different approaches, it has been shown that 74% and 83% of triploidies have a paternal origin mainly due to dispermy after in vivo and in vitro fertilization, respectively (Couillin et al. 1987). The small number of abortuses reported with a 69,XYY constitution reflects the poor developmental capacity of these embryos.

Tetraploidy

Tetraploidy represents 6% of the anomalies reported after in vivo fertilization (Boue and Boue 1976). Plachot et al. observed one case in their study (4.8%) (Plachot 1989). Shields et al. noted two cases (22.2%, one complete and one mosaic) (Shields et al. 1992), Roesler et al. reported one case (20%) in a quite small series (Roesler et al. 1989), while Barlow et al. observed none (Barlow et al. 1988). Stern et al. noted a fetal tetraploidy in 5.5% of chromosomally abnormal fetuses (7/128) (Stern et al. 1996).

The most common constitution is 92,XXXX. The fact that after in vivo fertilization all tetraploidies have an XXXX or XXYY sex chromosome constitution supports the hypothesis of a failure of cytokinesis during the first division of the diploid zygote or during early mitotic cleavage (Plachot 1989). After IVF tetraploid oocytes can be detected the day after insemination because of the presence of four pronuclei in the ooplasm. The two extra pronuclei can be either of paternal or maternal origin. When cultured for 7 days in vitro, none out of ten tetraploid embryos passed beyond the eight-cell stage (Plachot et al. 1988a). However, some of them are able to develop further in vivo as they are observed in first-trimester abortions and exceptionally at birth. In the Q strain of mice, 17% of tetraploid blastocysts are capable of sustaining postimplantation development (Snow 1975). Although polyspermy is another possible mechanism for both tetraploidy and triploidy, this is unlikely to be the cause of embryonic or fetal abnormalities in IVF, where the pronuclear stage of embryonic development is noted prior to transfer.

Structural Chromosomal Anomalies

A structural anomaly, namely a translocation, was observed by Plachot in 4.8% (Plachot 1989). The same incidence (3.8%) was reported after in vivo fertilization. In one-third of these cases the anomaly was transmitted from one of the parents, the others resulted from errors occurring during gametogenesis or at fertilization. It has been reported that 2.4% of couples entering an IVF programme have a chromosomal anomaly, half of these being a structural aberration (Hens et al. 1988). The incidence reaches 6% in couples with recurrent spontaneous abortions (Fortuny et al. 1988). The rate of chromosome imbalance in the general population is only 0.6% (Nielsen 1975). In the series of Shields et al. one case of inversion was observed (Shields et al. 1992).

Mosaics

Shields et al. found five sets of mosaic specimens in abortuses, while Roesler, Plachot and Barlow each reported one case of mosaics (Plachot 1989; Shields et al. 1992; Roesler et al. 1989; Barlow et al. 1988). The incidence of mosaics is higher in embryos in vitro before transfer (Munne et al. 1995). Therefore, one can assume that nearly all those embryos are either incapable of implantation or will be aborted preclinically.

Factors that Might Influence the Incidence of Chromosomal Anomalies

Effect of Ovarian Stimulation

Boue et al. found a significant increase in the level of chromosomal anomalies (mainly trisomies) among a series of 47 abortuses from women in whom ovulation had been induced (83%) when compared with a large sample of 1374 untreated women (60%) (Boue and Boue 1973; Boue et al. 1975). Plachot et al. found no difference in the incidence of chromosomal anomalies in abortuses of 19 patients treated with clomiphene/HMG (63%) when compared with 12 patients receiving GnRH analogues/HMG and two patients receiving HMG alone (67%) (Plachot 1989). After ovulation induction with gonadotropins, Asch et al. observed an abnormal karyotype in 72.0% of all cases of spontaneous abortion compared to 64.0% after spontaneous conceptions, which is in the same range (Asch et al. 1999).

More polyploid embryos were obtained in hormonally stimulated female rabbits and mice when compared with controls (Takagi and Sasaki 1976; Maudlin and Fraser 1977). Therefore, the authors concluded that superovulation treatment could have an adverse effect on the oocyte level by impairing polar body extrusion or cortical reactions, thus leading to polyploidy, rather than by a meiotic impairment leading to aneuploidy. In contrast, no increase in the incidence of aneuploidy or polyploidy has been reported by others in mice (Laing et al. 1984) or hamsters (Sengoku and Dukelow 1988).

Effect of ICSI

Meiotic disorders are frequent in infertile males and may increase with severe oligoasthenozoospermia. In these couples ICSI is usually applied. These patients produce spermatozoa with autosomal and sex disomies and diploid spermatozoa more often than fertile controls. Their contribution to spontaneous abortions depends on the production of trisomies, monosomies and triploidies. The most frequent sperm chromosome anomaly in infertile males is diploidy, originating from either a meiotic or a compromised testicular environment (Egozcue et al. 2000). Therefore, a higher rate of chromosomal anomalies might be expected in abortions occurring after ICSI. Hong et al. observed an abnormal karyotype in 57.8% of abortions occurring after ICSI, which is in the same range as the rate noted in abortions after IVF (62.0%) and after spontaneous conception (66.7%) (Hong et al. 1999). Coulam et al. compared the outcome of pregnancies after ICSI and after IVF with fresh and frozen ET and donor oocyte cycles and compared chromosomal findings after clinical pregnancy loss if a chromosomal analysis was available (Coulam et al. 1996). The rate of aneuploidy was 60% of all abortions occurring after ICSI, 50% after IVF, 33% after donor oocyte cycles and 50% after frozen ET. A polyploidy occurred in 13% of pregnancy losses after ICSI, in 25% after IVF, and in none after donor oocyte cycles or frozen ET. None of these differences was significant. Several studies looking for the incidence of abortions after an ICSI procedure are shown in Table 2.3.

In a recent study, the influences of sperm DNA decondensation – which is described as abnormal after ICSI – and of sperm diploidy rate on the incidence of chromosomal abnormalities in the offspring were compared (Sbracia et al. 2002). The authors concluded that it is much more likely that a high incidence of abnormal karyotypes in spermatozoa from men undergoing an ICSI treatment leads to the changed incidence in abnormal karyotypes in offspring as compared to changes in sperm DNA decondensation or the fertilization process after ICSI (Schröder et al. 2001; Ludwig et al. 2001b).

Effect of Parental Age

The effect of maternal age on the incidence of trisomies 13, 18 and 21, as well as of 47,XXX and 47,XXY conceptuses has been well documented (Boue et al. 1975; Boue and Boue 1976; Hook 1981). Earlier in development, the same effect has been reported in oocytes recovered for IVF (Plachot et al. 1988b), but not confirmed in a smaller series (Pellestor and Sele 1988). Conversely, no effect of maternal age has been shown for 45,X, triploid, tetraploid or translocated conceptuses (Boue and Boue 1976).

Plachot found a slight non-significant increase in the incidence of aneuploidy in abortuses from women above 38 years of age (75 %) when compared with younger patients (58 %), but no paternal effect was found, the incidence of chromosomal defects being 50 % for patients > 38 years of age and 71 % for younger patients (Plachot 1989). This is in good agreement with other studies (Boue and Boue 1976).

In mice, a doubling of the rate of aneuploidy has been demonstrated in old females when compared with control animals (Maudlin and Fraser 1978; Santalo et al. 1987) as well as a delay in cleavage associated with an increase in abnormal embryos (Gosden 1973). This is also confirmed by the FISH data of supernumerary embryos as mentioned above (Munne et al. 1995). In contrast, no effect of maternal age has been shown for 45,X, triploid, tetraploid or translocated conceptuses (Boue and Boue 1976; Munne et al. 1995).

Conclusion

The number of chromosome abnormalities in abortions following ART procedures seems not to be higher than following natural conception. These data, however, have mostly been derived by comparison with historical control groups. This may be the main explanation for the fact that some studies still indicate a slightly increased incidence of chromosomal abnormalities. On the other hand, other factors in an ART population, such as parental age and chromosome abnormalities of the parents, will contribute to this risk.

There are some conflicting data on the contribution of ovarian stimulation to chromosomal aberrations in the fetus. The main body of evidence, however, seems to show that in humans this effect is not present. This is perhaps also the reason why in ICSI pregnancies there is a higher incidence of gonosomal aberrations found. Male subfertility is associated with a higher rate of disomic spermatozoa, and it is this that results in the disturbance during meiotic division. However, more data are needed to give a final estimate of the actual risk of these men inducing a pregnancy with an chromosomally abnormal child.

4 Assisted Reproduction and Prenatal Diagnosis

Pia Wülfing, Michael Ludwig

As already mentioned, the ultimate goal of every infertility treatment is the birth of a healthy baby. Even if "healthy" cannot be defined, the prospective parents try everything to assure themselves that their child will not be affected by a serious disorder. Therefore, prenatal diagnostic procedures are of special clinical importance in pregnancies following assisted reproductive techniques (ART).

Prenatal diagnosis (PND) can be subdivided into invasive procedures, such as chorionic villous sampling (CVS) and amniocentesis (AC), and into non-invasive procedures, such as ultrasound and determination of serum markers. Invasive PND procedures, usually either CVS in the first trimester or AC in the second, can test the fetus for serious genetic defects. The defects, again, can be separated into two groups. First, defects for which there is a high risk if the parents are carriers of a mutation, and second, for example chromosome abnormalities, if there is an increased risk secondary to advanced maternal age or a chromosome abnormality associated with male factor infertility.

The chromosome abnormalities found in CVS can be divided into true fetal abnormalities and abnormalities confined to the placenta. CVS is estimated to carry a 1% risk and AC a 0.5% risk of subsequent spontaneous abortion. If the fetus is found to be affected, the couple is faced with the decision as to whether to terminate the pregnancy or to go on with it. Therefore, first of all, it is necessary to counsel the parents adequately as to whether there is any increased risk of abnormality. If not, there is no need to offer PND by another method as in spontaneously conceived pregnancies. Furthermore, as with every PND, the parents have to be counselled that not only a negative, but also a positive diagnosis, can be made – with the possibility of pregnancy termination. Finally, the risk of abortion following invasive PND has to be weighed against the chance of finding an abnormality. Here, again, data are needed to estimate the risk of abnormalities with the background of an ART procedure. Otherwise, sufficient counselling is not possible.

Invasive Prenatal Diagnosis

IVF and Prenatal Diagnosis

As early as 1979 Schlesselman et al. raised the concern about the risk of abnormalities due to in vitro fertilization (IVF), including oocyte collection, embryo culture and transfer. They suggested that an in vitro versus in vivo comparison might be made in the study of preimplantation embryos and spontaneous abortions, the results of AC, and the findings from fetal deaths and live births. They stressed that in vivo, 40% to 50% of implanted blastocysts are estimated to have a chromosome abnormality, over 99% of which are considered to be eliminated during the course of the pregnancy. Therefore, Schlesselman et al. assumed that in principle, the genetic evaluation of early spontaneous abortions would be more efficient than AC for detecting an increased risk of chromosome abnormalities at birth. They stated that a large number of births would be required to provide a definitive assessment of risk, unless IVF in humans strongly contradicts the experience in domestic animal reproduction, which suggests no increased risk of abnormalities at birth (Schlesselman 1979).

Since then, several studies have been published in which the outcome of pregnancies after more established ART procedures such as IVF, GIFT (gamete intrafallopian transfer), ZIFT (zygote intrafallopian transfer) and embryo cryopreservation has been investigated (e.g. Frydman et al. 1986; Rufat et al. 1994). The overall conclusions concerning these established techniques were that the frequency of cytogenetic abnormalities in fetuses and neonates from pregnancies after IVF was comparable to that found in the general population.

There are only a few studies available that document prenatal findings in the IVF populations. One of the earliest studies concerning IVF and PND was reported by Würfel et al. They reported their results of PND using AC in 63 pregnancies out of a cohort of 189 intact pregnancies (33%) after IVF performed between 1985 and 1987. In 75% of these pregnancies the indication for AC was advanced maternal age (> 35 years). In this study one case of trisomy 21 and four fetuses with structural chromosome abnormalities inherited from the parents without any clinical relevance were detected. The incidence of trisomy 21 was the same as in a normal population of women older than 35 years (1.6%). In contrast, the number of aberrations found in amniotic cultures in cases where it was identified additionally in one parent ($n = 4$) was above the average (7.9%). The results of this early study demonstrate that although the incidence of chromosome abnormalities in AC cultures is increased, the risk of relevant fetal chromosome aberrations is not higher in the IVF populations than in the normal population. This could be explained by the usually higher age and elevated risk of abnormal karyotypes in IVF-treated women (Würfel et al. 1992).

In't Veld et al. (1995a) carried out a retrospective study to investigate this problem of cytogenetic abnormalities in IVF pregnancies. In this study the cytogenetic abnormalities in a population of 252 fetuses from women with IVF pregnancies were recorded. All women were referred to the Institute of Human Genetics for PND between 1990 and 1994 due to advanced maternal age. Therefore, an enormous preselection of the study group must be kept in mind. In't Veld et al. compared the frequency of such abnormalities in IVF pregnancies with that in a control group of spontaneously conceived pregnancies. In the CVS group 11 chromosome abnormalities were found (13.8%): 6 fetal abnormalities and 5 confined placental mosaics (four trisomy 21 and three trisomy 7). In the AC group, identical rates were found (1.7%) in the IVF and control groups. In this study, the frequencies of both confined placental abnormalities and true fetal chromosome anomalies found by CVS in IVF pregnancies were significantly increased three- to fivefold ($P < 0.008$, $P < 0.04$, respectively). In contrast, the frequency of chromosome aberrations found by AC at 16–18 weeks of gestation was found to be similar to that in the controls (1.7%) (In't Veld et al. 1995b).

The difference between the results of AC and CVS may be explained in terms of several factors. For example, a high level of spontaneous abortions (29%) was reported in a group of IVF pregnancies with a maternal age over 35 years. Therefore, the fetal cytogenetic abnormalities may represent pregnancies that would have aborted spontaneously before AC at 16 weeks of gestation. It is concluded that in the late first trimester, but not in the early second trimester, IVF pregnancies are characterized by an increased frequency of cytogenetic abnormalities found at PND. The authors concluded that if an IVF pregnancy has an increased risk of spontaneous abortion due to a chromosome abnormality, PND by AC is the most suitable approach. This would avoid unnecessary interventions.

More recent results are provided by Van Golde et al. (1999). They performed PND in 1995 in 57 IVF and ICSI pregnancies. In each group (IVF or ICSI), 30% of couples chose invasive PND. The most frequent indication for PND was advanced maternal age, although couples were informed about a possible genetic risk of ICSI and therefore PND was offered in all cases. The mean maternal age was 33.67 ± 3.94 years (range 25–44 years) and the mean paternal age was 35.9 ± 5.38 years (25–69 years). An abnormal fetal karyotype was discovered by AC in two ICSI pregnancies. Small numbers and screening patients at high risk could be responsible for the high frequency of chromosome abnormalities (3.8%) (Van Golde et al. 1999).

The low uptake rate of PND in IVF patients is an interesting feature of the studies previously mentioned. This is also shown for different techniques in Table 4.1. Advanced maternal age was the main indication. As these women have a higher risk of abnormal karyotypes due to their age this could bias the results of fetal cytogenetic analysis. A possible explanation as to why people may decide against a chromosomal PND could be the risk of miscarriage, the present follow-up results and the unknown phenotypic consequence of some chromosome abnormalities. Therefore, Van Golde et al. concluded that male candidates for IVF/ICSI should have a detailed genetic work-up concerning family history, chromosome analysis and detection of genes involved in spermatogenesis, and should be offered genetic counselling. Following this counselling the couple could be offered a PND in some cases of genetic abnormalities.

In 1998 Schover et al. assumed that many couples undergoing IVF are at a higher risk of having a child with a genetic abnormality. In their study group of 55 sampled consecutive couples starting IVF, 67% had a genetic risk factor such as maternal age or possible abnormalities associated with severe male factor infertility. Despite counselling about these risks, 71% refused formal genetic work-up. However, 47% planned to have AC or CVS, although a triple test screening for fetal abnormalities was acceptable to 82% of couples. Those couples who would consider terminating a pregnancy if the fetus had a severe genetic abnormality were significantly more likely to opt for PND ($P < 0.01$). Socioeconomic

Table 4.1. Acceptance of invasive PND in pregnancies after ART (*n.a.* not available)

Reference	Year of publication	ART	Total no. of pregnancies	Invasive PND (karyotyped)	PND uptake rate (%)	Period of study
Hirsch et al.	1989	IVF	189	63	33	1985–1987
Wurfel et al.	1992	IVF	82	82	100[a]	1985–1989
Bonduelle et al.	1994	SUZI/ICSI	163	43	26	1991–1993
In't Veld et al.	1995	IVF	201	252	–[b]	1990–1994
In't Veld et al.	1995	ICSI	15	15	–[b]	1994–1995
Feichtinger et al.	1995	ICSI	61	7	11	n.a.
Liebaers et al.	1995	ICSI	n.a.	585	n.a.	n.a.
Wisanto et al.	1995	ICSI	320	238	74	1991–1994
Wisanto et al.	1996	ICSI	904	582	64.4	up to 1995
Bonduelle et al.	1996	ICSI	320	238	74	1991–1994
Palermo et al.	1996	ICSI	578	150	26	?
Tarlatzis	1996	ICSI	1321	362	27.4	1994
Testart et al.	1996	ICSI	83	108	100[c]	1994–1995
Van Opstal et al.	1997	ICSI	–[d]	71	–[d]	n.a.
Tarlatzis and Bili	1998	ICSI	2668	539	20.2	1995
Bonduelle et al.	1998c	ICSI	165	70	40	1991–1996
Meschede et al.	1998	ICSI	107	18	16.8	1995–1998
Van Golde et al.	1999	IVF/ICSI	190	57	30	1995
Bonduelle et al.	1999	ICSI	1987	1082	54.5	1992–1997
Causio et al.	1999	ICSI	301	74	25	1994
Loft et al.	1999	ICSI	642	183	28.5	1994–1997
Monni et al.	1999	ICSI	87	75	86.2	n.a.
Ludwig et al.	1999	ICSI	213	73	34.1	1994–1997
Westergaard et al.	1999, 2000	ART	1756	289	13.2	1994–1995
Tarlatzis and Bili	2000	ICSI	3855	566	14.7	1993–1995

[a] In this IVF program, AC was performed for all the pregnancies.
[b] All patients underwent invasive PND and all these data were evaluated at the Institute of Human Genetics, where the karyotyping was done.
[c] All ICSI pregnancies were karyotyped.
[d] All patients were referred for invasive PND due to advanced maternal age, ultrasound abnormalities or a previous child with abnormalities.

status and whether the infertility factor was male or female were shown not to be predictors of a couples' attitude (Schover et al. 1998).

Another recent report by Westergaard et al. (2000) provides data from the compulsory National Danish IVF Registry for the years 1994 and 1995. In 289 of 1800 ongoing pregnancies, invasive PND was performed (16%). Of these pregnancies, 207 with PND were achieved by IVF, 56 by ICSI and 20 after frozen embryo replacement. In the IVF pregnancies seven abnormal karyotypes were detected (3.4%).

Table 4.2. Results of PND in pregnancies after ART (*n.a.* not available)

Reference	ART	Invasive PND	Parental chromosome abnormalities	Maternal age (years) (n)	Fetal chromosome abnormalities	Inherited abnormalities	De novo abnormalities	Sex chromosome abnormalities	Abnormalities
Hirsch et al. 1989	IVF	63	46,XY,15p+; 46,XY,16qh+; 46,XX,inv(7)(p12q22); 47,XX,mar+;	>35 (n = 47)	5 (7.9%)	4 (6.3%)	1 (1.6%)	0	47,XX,+2; 46,XY,15p+; 46,XY,16qh+; 46,XX,inv(7)(p12q22); 47,XX,mar+
Wurfel et al. 1992	IVF	82	46,XY,15p+ (male); 46,XY,16qh+ (female); 46,XY,inv(7)(p12q22)(m); 47,XX,+mar (female); 46,XY,inv(9)	>35 (n = 56)	6 (7.3%)	4 (4.9%)	2 (2.4%)	0	47,XX,+2; 46,XY,15+; 46,XY,16qh+; 46,xx,inv(7)(p12q22); 47,XX,+mar; 47,XX,+21
Bonduelle et al. 1994	SUZI/ICSI	43	46,XY,inv(1)(p22p23.1) (male)	>35 (n = 11)	1 (1.8%)	1 (2.3%)	0	0	46,XY,inv(1)(p22p23.1)

Table 4.2 (continued)

Reference	ART	Invasive PND	Parental chromosome abnormalities	Maternal age (years) (n)	Fetal chromosome abnormalities	Inherited abnormalities	De novo abnormalities	Sex chromosome abnormalities	Abnormalities
In't Veld et al. 1995	IVF	252	n.a.	–[a]	14 (5%)	n.a.	n.a.	4 (1.6%)	45,X/46,X, dic(Y)(q11)/46, X,del(Y)(q11); 47,XY,+2; 47,XYY; 47,XX,+2; 47,XY, +21; 46,XX/47,XX, +21(2/28); 45, X/46,XY (12/22); 46,XY/47,XY, +7/48,XY,+7, +13 (8/2/40); 46,XY/47,XY, +7 (11/21); 45, X/46,XX (2/18); 47,XX,+7
In't Veld et al. 1995	ICSI	15	n.a.	–[a]	6 (40%)	n.a.	n.a.	6 (40%)	47,XXY; 47,XXY; 45,X/46,X.dic(Y) (q11)/46.X.del(Y) (Q11); 45,X; 45,X
Feichtinger et al. 1995	ICSI	7	n.a.	n.a.	0	0	0	0	0
Liebaers et al. 1995	ICSI	585	n.a.	n.a.	6 (1%)	n.a.	n.a.	5 (0.8%)	47,XXY; 47,XXY; 47,XXX; 47, XYY; 46,XX/47,XXX; 47,XY+21

[a] "Advanced maternal age" (exact age not given).

Reference	Method	n		Age					Karyotype findings
Wisanto et al. 1995; Bonduelle et al. 1996	ICSI	238	46,XY,inv(1)(p22p23.3) (2 male); 46,XY, inv(5)(p13q13) (male); 47,XX, +inv dup(15p) (male); 45,XY, t(14q21q) (male); 45,XX,t(11;17) (q23;q25) (female)	>35 (n = 75)	5 (2.1%)	4 (1.7%)	0	1 (0.4%)	46,XX/47, XXX(1/13); 46,XY,inv(1) (p22p23.3); 46,XY,inv(5) (p13q13); 47,XX, +inv dup(15p); 47,XX, +inv dup(15p)
Tarlatzis 1996	ICSI	362	n.a.	n.a.	8 (2.2%)	n.a.	n.a.	n.a.	n.a.
Testart et al. 1996	ICSI	116	46,XY,t(13;14); 45,XY,t(13;14) (5 male); 46,XY, t(3;20)(q13q13); 46,XY,t(15;19) (p12p11); 46,XY, inv2(p11;q13); 46,XY,inv2(p11;q13); 47,XY+mar bisat; 46,XX,t(3;9)(q13;q34); 46,XX,t(8;12)(q23;q32) 46,XX,inv14(q23;q32)	Mean 33.1 ± 0.2	5 (4.3%)	5 (4.3%)	5 (4.3%)	0	46,XY,t(13;14) (2 carriers); 46,XY,inv2 (p11q13); 46,XX,inv14 (q23;q32) (2 carriers)
Van Opstal et al. 1997	ICSI	71	6 male (sex), 2 female (autosomal)	>35 (n = 25)	9 (12.7%)	0	9 (12.7%)	6 (8.4%)	47,XXY; 47,XXY; 45,X0; 45,X0; 45,X/46,XY; 46,X,del(Y)(q11)/ 46,X,idic(Y) (q11)/45,X; 2 cases of trisomy 18; trisomy 21
Tarlatzis and Bili 1998	ICSI	539	n.a.	n.a.	11(2%)	n.a.	n.a.	n.a.	n.a.

Table 4.2 (continued)

Reference	ART	Invasive PND	Parental chromosome abnormalities	Maternal age (years) (n)	Fetal chromosome abnormalities	Inherited abnormalities	De novo abnormalities	Sex chromosome abnormalities	Abnormalities
Bonduelle et al. 1998	ICSI	70	All tested parents (29%) normal	n.a.	2 (5.8%)	0	0	2 (2.9%)	47,XXY; 47,XXY
Meschede et al. 1998	ICSI	18	5	> 35 (n = 22)	1 (5.5%)	n.a	n.a.	n.a.	Unbalanced translocation
Van Golde et al. 1999	IVF/ICSI	57	45,XY,t(13q,14q)	Mean 33.67	2 (3.5%)	1	1	1	45,XY,t(13q,14q); 45,X0
Bonduelle et al. 1999	ICSI	1082	n.a.	Mean 33.3	28 (2.78%)	10 (0.9%)	18 (1.7%)	9 (0.8%)	*De novo:* sex chromosomes (n = 9): 45,X; 46,XX/47,XXX; 3 cases of 47,XXX; 4 cases of 47,XXY; autosomal trisomies (n = 5): 3 cases of 47,XY +21; trisomy 21 47,XY(+18). *Inherited:* balanced (n = 9): 46,XY, inv(1)(p22p23.1); 46,XY,inv(5) (p13q13); 46,XX,t(14;15); 46,XX,t(13;14); 2 cases of 46,XX, +invdup(15p);

Reference	Method	n	Parental chromosome abnormalities	Maternal age				Fetal chromosome abnormalities	
Causio et al. 1999	ICSI	74	Male (n = 9): 46,XY,t(5;8)(q23; p23); 46,XY,t(6;11) (q26q22); 45,XY,t(14;21); 45,XY,t(13;14); 45,XY,t(21;22); 45,XY,t(14;21); 45,XY,t(13;14); 45,XY,t(13;14); 45,XY,t(13;14); female (n = 2): 46,XX,t(8;11) (q23;q25); 46,XX, t(6;18)(q16;q23)	Fetal abnormalities: mean 30.5 ± 3.5; no abnormalities: mean 33.9 ± 4.1	3 (4%)	2 (2.7%)	1 (1.4%)	47,XY,+13; 2 male fetuses with balanced chromosome abnormalities	45,XY,t(13;14); 45,XX,t(14;15); 45,XY,t(13q;14q); unbalanced (n = 1): 46,XY, t(14;21)+21
Loft et al. 1999	ICSI	209	T(9;22)pat	32.1	7 (3.3%)	1 (0.5%)	6 (2.9%)	Trisomy 13; trisomy 18; 2 cases of trisomy 21; unbalanced: t(17;22); triploidy; de novo: t(9;22)pat	
Monni et al. 1999	ICSI	75	n.a.	35	n.a.	n.a.	0	Trisomy 21	
Westergaard et al. 1999	ART	289	n.a.	>35 (57.6%)	10 (3.5%)	n.a.	n.a.	n.a.	
Tarlatzis and Bili 2000	ICSI	566	n.a.	n.a.	12 (2.1%)	n.a.	n.a.	n.a.	

Furthermore, PND revealed three chromosome aberrations in the ICSI pregnancies and none after frozen embryo replacement. Compared with the normal population, the incidence of chromosome aberrations was elevated. As already mentioned, this could be explained by the higher age of IVF-treated women which generally causes a higher risk of abnormal karyotypes (Westergaard et al. 2000).

The overall conclusions concerning these established techniques is that the frequency of cytogenetic abnormalities in fetuses and neonates from pregnancies after IVF is comparable to that in the general population, especially when certain risk factors of the population undergoing an ART procedure is taken into account. Therefore, an IVF origin of a pregnancy is generally not considered to be sufficient indication for invasive PND (Rizk et al. 1991a; Testart et al. 1992). An overview regarding abnormalities in PND after IVF, as well as after other techniques, is shown in Table 4.2.

ICSI and Prenatal Diagnosis

The major breakthrough in the treatment of male factor infertility was the introduction of ICSI to reproductive medicine in the early 1990s (Palermo et al. 1992). This has provided the possibility to achieve high fertilization and pregnancy rates for couples with severe male factor infertility and therefore the chance to conceive their own biological children (Van Steirteghem et al. 1993). Men with severe oligospermia or azoospermia can now pass their genes on to their progeny, an event that might not have been possible for them just a few years ago. This has also improved the prospects of couples with multiple failure in conventional IVF.

Regarding the genetic background of these men, at least three different things have to be considered. First, it is well known that there is about a tenfold increased risk of a chromosome abnormality – structural or numerical – in men with oligozoospermia (Meschede et al. 1998b). This risk correlates negatively with the number of sperms in the ejaculate, reaching a 30-fold increased risk in men with azoospermia. Therefore, a chromosome analysis before starting an ICSI cycle is mandatory. Second, the risk of obstructive azoospermia in cases of congenital bilateral absence of the vas deferens (CBAVD) is linked to mutations in the cystic fibrosis transmembrane regulator (CFTR) gene which is responsible for autosomally recessive transmitted cystic fibrosis. Meanwhile, it is accepted that CBAVD is a minor form of cystic fibrosis and therefore needs genetic counselling and a genetic work-up (Chillon et al. 1995). Finally, there is a substantial risk of Y-chromosome microdeletions in men suffering from severe oligozoospermia or azoospermia (Reijo et al. 1996). Patients have to be counselled about this, since a microdeletion means that every son born after ICSI will also suffer from male subfertility with a high probability in the future (Page et al. 1999). On the other hand, these deletions will not cause any harm to the general health of these men and screening for Y-chromosome microdeletions might not be sensible in every case, especially since not every genetic background risk for male subfertility alone can be excluded – since most genes are not known yet. However, couples have to be counselled that there remains a genetic risk of transmission of male factor infertility – even when testing for the most severe conditions has proved negative.

In this context, Bofinger et al. reported that approximately 13.7% of infertile men with azoospermia and 4.6% with oligozoospermia have a coexistent chromosome abnormality (Bofinger et al. 1999). Although the ICSI procedure appears safe so far, for men whose infertility is linked to genetic conditions, predicting the potential effects on their offspring remains an unprecedented challenge. Therefore, PND procedures have extra value in ICSI pregnancies, as compared to pregnancies after conventional IVF, in which most often a female factor instead of male factor infertility will be present.

Based on the discussion above, the current policy regarding PND in ICSI pregnancies is not uniform, as has been shown by a review of the literature. In two Belgian centres, CVS or AC was initially a mandatory part of the treatment protocol (Bonduelle et al. 1994; Govaerts et al. 1995), although uptake rates far below 100% were reported. Two Swedish groups offered AC on a non-compulsory basis, and prenatal chromosome tests were performed in only 33–41% of their ICSI pregnancies (Bui and Wramsby 1996; Wennerholm et al. 1996). Testart et al. (1996) in France karyotyped all their ICSI pregnancies although it is not entirely clear from their report whether this was a general policy or only applied to pregnancies of patients with abnormal karyotypes (Testart et al. 1996). The Austrian group of Feichtinger et al. (1995) described a low acceptance of invasive PND in their ICSI population of only 11% (Feichtinger et al. 1995). In Germany, Ludwig et al. reported that about 30% of their patients underwent invasive PND (Ludwig et al. 1999c). The policy of another German group was to offer an AC or another invasive procedure on a voluntary basis. The uptake rate for invasive tests was low, although many women had an indication independent of ICSI (Meschede et al. 1998c). Most patients in this population preferred non-invasive options. Meschede et al. concluded that their pretherapeutic genetic counselling session had a reassuring effect for many patients treated with ICSI, and that consequently they were less anxious about abnormalities in their pregnancy (Table 4.1).

Concerning this, Geipel et al. (1999) reported a decreasing rate of invasive PND due to the introduction of what they call "genetic sonography" at their centre in 1995. The rate of invasive PND was 74% in 1995, 48% in 1996, 36% in 1997 and 19% in 1998 (Geipel et al. 1999). Their data confirmed those of Meschede et al. (1998c) who showed that 82% of patients getting pregnant after ICSI strongly favoured non-invasive prenatal testing, if they had the option and were counselled appropriately.

However, some studies have revealed a significantly increased risk for chromosome abnormalities in pregnancies conceived through ICSI. The subject of much discussion are the results reported by In't Veld et al., who expressed concerns about the genetic risks for the offspring of ICSI pregnancies. They reported a very limited series, in which 6 sex chromosome anomalies were found out of 15 ICSI pregnancies tested by CVS due to advanced maternal age. Consequently, in this series the rate of chromosome anomalies was about 40% (In't Veld et al. 1995a). This figure is much higher than those reported by other groups. A possible explanation for this might be that the series of In't Veld et al. were women who had been referred to their Institute of Human Genetics for PND, as has already been mentioned above. This means an enormous preselection. Therefore, this figure does not correctly represent the true situation and is rather a result of small numbers and of preselection of patients.

The type of chromosome aberrations observed in this series of ICSI pregnancies is in line with the data of Van Opstal et al. (1997) who reported the results of prenatal cytogenetic analysis. Of 71 fetuses conceived by ICSI, 9 chromosome aberrations were detected, i.e. an incidence of 12.7%. These chromosome anomalies included six sex chromosome abnormalities and three autosomal trisomies. Molecular analysis was performed using polymorphic microsatellite markers to determine the parental origin of the deleted or supernumerary chromosome. Six cases of sex chromosome aberrations were proven to be of paternal origin while the two trisomic cases were of maternal origin. The high incidence of chromosome anomalies could also be explained in this study by a preselected cohort of patients, as at least 29 of 71 PNDs were performed due to advanced maternal age, sonographic anomalies, and a history of previous children born with malformations (Van Opstal et al. 1997).

Another retrospective study of 437 pregnancies after ICSI was performed by Palermo et al. (1996). Only 150 of their patients (26%) wished to undergo invasive PND which showed a high rate of 11 fetuses with chromosome aberrations (7.3%) (Palermo et al. 1996).

Loft et al. (1999) performed a national cohort study including all clinical pregnancies obtained after ICSI registered in Denmark between 1994 and 1997 at 13 fertility clinics. The mean age of the women was 32.1 years. PND resulted in 209 karyotypes (28.5% uptake) with seven (3.3%) chromosome aberrations. Of these, six were major chromosome abnormalities (2.9%) and one was an inherited structural chromosome aberration (0.5%). However, no sex chromosome aberrations were detected (Loft et al. 1999).

Other data on PND and ICSI are provided by the report on the activities of the ESHRE Task Force on ICSI (Tarlatzis 1996; Tarlatzis and Bili 1998, 2000). The results of prenatal screening in 362 (27.4%), 539 (20.2%), and 566 (14.7%) pregnancies, respectively, conceived by ICSI were recorded. In this sample, invasive PND revealed 8 (2.2%), 11 (2%), and 12 (2.1%) abnormal fetal karyotypes, respectively. Compared to the general population, these figures appear slightly higher than expected (Jacobs et al. 1992). However, it should be taken into account that the size of the basic sample of this database remains to be elucidated. It is also unclear, whether the reported chromosome aberrations of the ESHRE Task Force include aberrations only among live births or also those among stillbirths and terminated pregnancies. Furthermore, the database does not clarify whether each participating centre reported chromosome anomalies and provided a follow-up of pregnancy course and children. Another interesting point is that Tarlatzis et al. also included benign structural aberrations such as inversions or translocations, and therefore the data are not strictly comparable with those of other groups. These problems of a multinational register also impact on other aspects of ART pregnancies – such as those discussed in Chapter 7.

One study that provides prospective data on the collection of karyotypes in children born after ICSI is available (Aboulghar et al. 2001). In this prospective, controlled study from Egypt, 430 babies born after ICSI from 320 pregnancies were included. As a control group 430 babies from 413 naturally conceived pregnancies were included. An abnormal karyotype was found in 15 babies from the ICSI group (3.5%) and in none of the controls. This difference was significant with an odds ratio of 31.0 (95% confidence interval 1.86–516.45). However, some criticism of these data must be mentioned. Regarding the study design, it is not clear how many children in total were conceived during the study period. Only those pregnancies that were seen by the obstetricians of the university were included. This may have resulted in a preselection of problematic pregnancies. Furthermore, only in 6 out of 15 abnormal karyotypes could the parental karyotype be established. In two out of these there was an abnormal paternal karyotype, reducing the incidence from 3.5% to 3.0% of non-inherited cases. Since inheritance in the remaining cases cannot be excluded, the true prevalence of an abnormal karyotype after ICSI at birth may be in the range of 2.3% to 2.5%, which should no longer be significantly different from the controls. To conclude, as the authors themselves mention, these data should be used for counselling of couples who undergo ICSI, and show only a minimal increase – if any – in the rate of abnormal karyotypes at birth (Aboulghar et al. 2001).

The only extensive prospective follow-up study that allows a realistic estimation of the potential risks of ICSI was reported by Bonduelle et al. (2002). A total of 2889 children born after ICSI between 1992 and 1999 were included. The authors provide data on PND, congenital malformations, growth parameters and developmental milestones up to the age of 2 years, as well as on genetic counselling of the parents. Invasive PND was performed in 1437 fetuses and 42 chromosome aberrations (2.9%) were detected (Table 4.3). In detail, 23 abnormal karyotypes were de novo (1.6%), 9 of which were sex chromosome aberrations. Furthermore, 19 karyotypes (1.32%) with inherited structural aberrations were detected. Of these, 15 structural aberrations were transmitted from the father. The mean maternal age of 32.7 years would correspond to a value of 0.3% chromosome aberrations in PND in a normal population (Ferguson-Smith 1983). Therefore, the increased incidence of chromosome aberrations in these ICSI patients cannot be explained by maternal age alone. In this study a slight

Table 4.3. Abnormal results of PND in 1437 fetuses after ICSI (data according to Bonduelle et al. 2002)

Type of chromosome abnormality	Number	Percentage
De novo	23	1.60
Autosomal	14	0.92
Numerical	6	0.46
Structural	8	0.56
Gonosomal	9	0.68
Inherited	19	1.32

increase (about threefold) of de novo sex chromosome aberrations was proven (0.63%), whereas the percentage of aberrations in a neonatal population has been reported to be 0.19% (Jacobs et al. 1992), 0.2%, and up to 0.23% (Nielsen and Wohlert 1991). Whether this difference was statistically significant or not is not mentioned in the report of this study. However, this increase might probably be directly linked to the characteristics of the infertile men treated rather than to the ICSI procedure itself. However, all de novo gonosomal aberrations were found in pregnancies of couples with extreme oligoasthenoteratozoospermia. The observed increase in autosomal chromosome aberrations can partly be explained by an increase in trisomies, linked with higher maternal age. Bonduelle et al. also found a higher number of inherited aberrations than in the general population, which was predictable for the individual couple. In all but four of these, the father was the carrier of the structural anomaly.

The authors also pointed out that during the genetic counselling before the ICSI procedure they included a number of couples with an increased risk for monogenic disorders – estimated for 78 children – because they wished to undergo preimplantation genetic diagnosis (Bonduelle et al. 1999). There were 27 children at risk due to karyotype anomalies in their parents, especially of fathers with either gonosomal aberrations or structural abnormalities (4.8%). This percentage is much higher than the expected figure of 0.5% in the general population (Jacobs et al. 1992), and may be explained by severe male factor infertility present in the population of ICSI patients.

In conclusion, there appears to be some risk of transmitting chromosome aberrations of de novo, mainly sex chromosome, aberrations and of transmitting fertility problems to the offspring. In contrast, these observations on a limited number of children do not suggest a higher incidence of diseases linked to imprinting, nor do they suggest a higher incidence of congenital malformations in children born after ICSI.

After these findings were published, the question was raised as to whether the ICSI technique per se has effects on the children born as it bypasses the never-proven selection of spermatozoa by the zona pellucida and the oolemma (Butler 1995). However, there is as yet no evidence which supports the hypothesis that fertilizing spermatozoa are somehow selected and that only morphologically normal spermatozoa can achieve fertilization (Yanagimachi 1995). Another speculation is that the genetic defects responsible for sperm impairment could be passed to the male offspring. Several reports concerning these issues have been published.

The problem that, apart from abnormalities arising de novo, abnormal karyotypes may be directly derived from predisposing parental aberrations has also been extensively discussed (Meschede et al. 1998a). These authors provide data from their prospective study in which 7.6% couples out of 868 were diagnosed with an aberrant karyotype. Their data are interesting in particular because more than 70% of the chromosome abnormalities were found among the women, although male factor infertility was twice as common as female factor infertility in their cohort. Therefore, the authors recommend that due to the high rate of abnormal karyotypes in females, not only the males, but both partners should be routinely karyotyped prior to ICSI. This finding of a high prevalence of chromosome aberrations in female partners of couples undergoing ICSI has been confirmed by others (Scholtes et al. 1998; Peschka et al. 1999). This is in contrast to the widespread opinion that genetic defects responsible for paternal sperm impairment can in particular be passed to the male offspring. These aberrations, which often appear as mosaics, apparently do not compromise the fertility of these women (Sonntag et al. 2001).

Very early data concerning the problem of a genetic risk in subfertile men were provided in 1975 (Chandley et al. 1975). At that time results of chromosome analysis in subfertile men were published, and they showed an increased incidence of chromosome aberrations in this group of males (2.2%) compared with the rate of 1% of karyotype abnormalities in the general male population. Furthermore, in cases of low sperm count or azoospermia, Retief et al. described a frequency of chromosome aberrations as high as 7–14% (Retief et al. 1984), and this has been confirmed by others (Bofinger et al. 1999). As Koulischer et al. have discussed, current IVF techniques including ICSI using ejaculated, epididymal or testicular spermatozoa clearly prevent any selection of spermatozoa with an abnormal karyotype either by the operator or by the oocyte (Koulischer et al. 1997). According to the widely admitted concept of gamete selection, pregnancies following ICSI, when compared to natural fertilization, therefore present a higher risk of genetic anomalies. However, this concept has not yet been proven.

Although follow-up studies have not shown an increased risk of malformation (Wisanto et al. 1995; Palermo et al. 1996; Wennerholm et al. 1996; Bonduelle et al. 1996a, 1999; Tarlatzis and Bili 1998), the genetic implications of ICSI are still not fully understood. The previously described high prevalence of structural and numerical chromosome aberrations among severely infertile men treated with ICSI is the basis of the concerns about the genetic risks. Several authors have postulated that patients with severe infertility could therefore be carriers of genetic lesions that might result in an increased prevalence of heritable disorders among their offspring (Cummins and Jequier 1994; Engel et al. 1996; Kurinczuk and Bower 1997; Rappaport et al. 1998).

To investigate the genetic safety of ICSI and therefore to evaluate the general genetic constitution of couples who need reproductive technology to procreate, Meschede et al. (2000) determined the frequency of potentially heritable non-reproductive diseases in 621 infertile couples and their first-degree relatives. There was a slightly higher prevalence of potentially heritable non-reproductive disorders in infertile patients than in controls (1.9% versus 0.9%; $P = 0.015$). In contrast, such diseases were less prevalent in their families than in the fertile couples' families. Meschede et al. conclude that their data do not support the notion that their familial genetic background predisposes children born after ICSI to malformations or other non-reproductive genetic diseases (Meschede et al. 2000). However, these data reflect the increased genetic risk in these couples.

In the same context, Meschede et al. (2000) examined the recurrence pattern of infertility in infertile couples' families in the same cohort characterized previously (Meschede et al. 2000). In their patient population, 6.4% of infertile couples had a fertility problem with a definite genetic basis which demonstrates a distinct pattern of familial aggregation only in infertile men. The infertile couples had fewer siblings compared to the fertile controls, which could be explained by suboptimal fertility among the infertile couples' parents as well. The authors concluded that genetic factors play a substantial role in the pathogenesis of human infertility, but that in particular only male factor infertility should be considered to have a major familial component. They assumed that male factor infertility may be a potentially heritable condition and that the recurrence risk for infertility in the offspring of couples treated with ICSI might be substantial. Evaluation of the exact risk of ICSI for the offspring, although desirable, seems to be nearly impossible. A prospective randomized trial would be necessary, but this cannot avoid the difficulty, for example, that it is impossible to compare an ICSI population with a fertile population. Assessment of the exact risk of ICSI and determination of whether the ICSI technique per se or the complex problem of male infertility is responsible for the increased incidence of chromosome aberrations in ICSI children would also require karyotyping of all pregnancies which would be ethically questionable.

Review of available data also shows that various groups have described a higher prevalence of gonosomal aberrations after ICSI which may be due to the problem of male infertility itself. The nature of sex chromosome abnormalities of the offspring after ICSI is still unclear. In this regard, it has to be established whether maternal or paternal meiotic errors are involved. The effects of the ICSI procedure on oocyte meiosis would have to be investigated in the case of a maternal origin, although it is unclear by what mechanism sex chromosome abnormalities could be induced. More likely are defects of paternal origin. A predominantly paternal origin of the abnormalities could indicate that the specific male fertility problems that led to ICSI may in some cases be accompanied by an increased incidence of sex chromosome abnormalities in sperm cells.

The impact of gonosomal aberrations on children's' health differs from that of, for example, autosomal trisomies. Meschede and Horst (1997) pointed out that gonosomal aberrations are not usually associated with malformations or other major congenital handicaps and discussed the developmental prognosis of individuals who carry a sex chromosome anomaly. They also emphasized that mental retardation does not occur more often in these individuals as in genetically normal controls. Therefore, the authors advice that in cases of a prenatally diagnosed gonosomal aberration, unbiased and detailed counselling concerning the developmental perspectives should be provided. They emphasize that the prognostic significance of a prenatally diagnosed sex chromosome anomaly should be neither under- nor overestimated (Meschede and Horst 1997).

As there seems to be no doubt that children born after ICSI carry an increased risk of infertility, even in cases of a normal paternal karyotype, Testart et al. recommended that PND be performed and all conceptuses be karyotyped to limit the genetic risk for infertility (Testart et al. 1996). This would guarantee detecting aneuploidies resulting from either paternal mosaicism (Persson et al. 1996) or abnormal chromosome pairing during spermatogenesis (Martin 1996). However, it is not possible to rule out the risk of infertility problems in offspring after either ART procedure, since most genetic causes are still unknown. Furthermore, couples undergoing ICSI will not be convinced of the necessity for invasive PND by the possible prospect of infertility in their children. However, although PND is assumed to be safe in ICSI pregnancies (Aytoz et al. 1998), there remains anxiety in patients regarding invasive PND that may cause low uptake rates described earlier in this chapter. Bonduelle et al. (1996a) assumed that ethical considerations could be a possible explanation for the patients scepticism concerning invasive PND.

Another reason is that patients consider the risk of miscarriage after fertility treatment too high. In fact, Bonduelle et al. reported three late abortions (two after AC and one after CVS) among 238 tested pregnancies (1.2%) that could be attributed to a PND procedure (Bonduelle et al. 1996a). This is comparable to the general population with regard to singletons (Tabor et al. 1986; Jahoda et al. 1991; Hanson et al. 1985) and twin pregnancies (Pergament et al. 1992; Wapner et al. 1993; De Catte et al. 1996). It is interesting that on the one hand, the expected risk of the test procedure from the limited data of Bonduelle et al. and from figures in the general population are 0.5–1%, and on the other hand the risk of a chromosome abnormality in the ICSI population in the described study was 1/293 (0.3%). This rate of chromosome abnormalities was approximately what could be expected in regularly conceived children and a mean maternal age of 32.1 years. One might therefore argue that as many ART centres routinely karyotype both partners to evaluate the general risk an additional risk from prenatal test procedures could be avoided if PND were performed only in cases of parental structural aberrations. If any structural aberrations were found, the risk for a non-balanced anomaly would be real and selective counselling would be possible.

The policy of Meschede et al. (1998) was to offer invasive PND on a voluntary basis. The uptake rate for invasive PND was low (17%) although 54% of women had an indication independent of ICSI (Meschede et al. 1998c). Meschede et al. assumed that the pretherapeutic genetic counselling may have had a reassuring effect for many patients treated with ICSI, and that consequently they were less anxious about abnormalities in their pregnancy. The authors stated that if patients pregnant through ICSI have the option to choose freely between invasive and non-invasive prenatal tests, they strongly favour the latter. Concerning the anxiety of patients regarding invasive PND, Meschede et al. suggested that the potential risk of an abortion induced by the invasive procedure may be the reason for low uptake rates. The authors do not consider the presumably increased prevalence (1%) of sex chromosome anomalies as an unequivocal reason for an invasive prenatal test as most of these aberrations are clinically benign. Therefore, couples treated with ICSI should, as others, have the opportunity to choose their options regarding PND in accordance with their own goals and values.

Non-invasive Prenatal Diagnosis

There are very few data published about ART and non-invasive PND. One of the basic reports concerning the discussion as to whether invasive or non-invasive

PND should preferably be performed in pregnancies after IVF/ICSI is that by Meschede et al. (1998). They reported the strong preference for non-invasive PND in 107 patients pregnant through ICSI between 1995 and 1998. In their centre of those patients counselled about PND, 65 had already received genetic counselling prior to the treatment (group 1) and 42 had not attended their clinic before (group 2). Only 18 of these patients (17%) opted for invasive PND procedures including AC or fetal blood sampling, whereas 87 patients (82%) opted for non-invasive PND. The preference for non-invasive procedures was stronger in group 1 (94%) than in group 2 (65%). Meschede et al. concluded that if patients pregnant through ICSI have the option to choose freely between invasive and non-invasive PND, they strongly favour the latter. They suggested that the potential risk of an abortion induced by the invasive procedures may be the reason for the anxiety of patients regarding invasive PND and this may have led to the low uptake rates (Meschede et al. 1998c).

Ultrasound

Over the last decade, both maternal age and the use of ART and drugs for the induction of ovulation have risen. This has resulted in a dramatic increase in multiple pregnancies at high risk for specific prenatal problems (Snijders et al. 1996). In this context, regular and established screening modalities for pregnancies have been shown to be ineffective in multiple gestations. For example, maternal serum screening in twin pregnancies exhibits a lower detection rate (Neveux et al. 1996). Additionally, while an affected co-twin may be indicated via screening techniques, identification of the fetus concerned has been demonstrated to be difficult. Furthermore, maternal serum marker concentrations may be affected by ART per se. On the other hand, ultrasound measurements (biparietal diameter, crown rump length) show a very good correlation with the estimated gestational age from IVF pregnancies with correlation coefficients ranging from 0.97 up to 0.99 (Tunon et al. 2000). Therefore, ultrasound is a much more reliable technique than serum markers.

Maymon et al. (1999) examined the feasibility of nuchal translucency (NT) measurement in higher order multiple gestations achieved by ART. A group of 79 fetuses – 1 patient with septuplets, 3 patients with quadruplets, 20 patients with triplets – were matched with 79 singleton controls. In this study NT measurements were feasible for both study and control fetuses, which exhibited similar NT measurements for the 5th, 50th, and 95th percentiles. Also mean NT thickness was similar in both groups. Maymon et al. could not detect any chromosome abnormalities prenatally in either group, and, of those infants who had no karyotyping, no traits were observed that warranted chromosome analysis. Since there is no other effective screening modality for these pregnancies, as maternal serum markers are less efficient for chromosome screening and mothers are worried about any invasive PND procedure, it seems reasonable to recommend NT measurement for PND (Maymon et al. 1999).

Geipel et al. (1999) investigated genetic sonography as the preferred option for PND in patients with pregnancies following ICSI. In this series, 153 patients pregnant after ICSI between 1995 and 1998 were screened by NT measurement (cut-off level > 3 mm). The screened 189 fetuses were differentiated into 22 singletons (80.3%), 23 twins (14.5%) and 8 triplet pregnancies (5.2%). Of these, 87 fetuses were scanned at 10–14 weeks of gestation. Six fetuses showed a NT that exceeded 3 mm. Consequently, in these cases prenatal chromosome analysis was performed and showed a normal karyotype. The remaining cohort of 102 fetuses were screened via second trimester sonography. In 88 of the 102 a normal scan was demonstrated, while an abnormal scan was present in 14. Altogether, in this study, two inherited numerical and structural chromosome anomalies in clinically healthy children at birth (1%) and four major malformations among all live-born children and late abortions (2.1%) were observed. The postnatally confirmed malformation rate of 2.1% (4/189) is comparable to the normal malformation rate. The authors recommend that, especially in women of advanced reproductive age with a long history of infertility, detailed genetic sonography may be a reasonable and highly accepted alternative to avoid invasive procedures.

Serum Markers for Prenatal Diagnosis

As discussed above, maternal serum marker concentrations may be affected by various ARTs. Moreover, regular screening modalities have been shown to be ineffective in twin and higher order pregnancies, the number of which is increasing over recent years due to ART.

Ribbert et al. reported their experience with maternal serum screening for fetal Down syndrome in a series of 67 IVF pregnancies (1991–1994) (Ribbert et al. 1996). A group of 4732 spontaneously conceiving patients served as controls. The pregnant patients' serum was screened between 15 and 20 weeks of gestation for alpha-fetoprotein (AFP) and human chorionic gonadotropin (hCG) for detection of Down syndrome. AFP levels were significantly lower (mean difference log MOM 0.053, $P < 0.01$) while hCG levels were significantly higher (mean difference log MOM 0.110, $P < 0.01$) in IVF patients than in controls. Altogether, 22 of 67 IVF patients (32.8%) were proven to be screen-positive. Of these, 17 decided to undergo AC which detected normal fetal karyotypes in all of them. Newborns of the other five screen-positive patients who refused AC appeared healthy and without traits that warranted chromosome analysis. The authors could not explain the fact that AFP levels were significantly lower and hCG levels significantly higher in pregnant IVF patients. The results of this study stress that caution in the interpretation of serum screening results in IVF pregnancies is essential, because unless AFP and hCG values are adjusted for in IVF pregnancies, the risk of Down syndrome in IVF pregnancies will be overestimated.

A similar analysis was performed by Barkai et al., who examined maternal serum AFP, hCG, and unconjugated oestriol levels in 1632 pregnant women following ovulation induction and 327 following IVF (Barkai et al. 1996). In accordance with the data of Ribbert et al., the results showed a highly statistically significant increase in hCG and reduction in oestriol among those patients with ovulation induction. There was no overall change in the median AFP level, but this masked a significant increase when treatment was with clomiphene and a significant decrease when human menopausal gonadotropin was used. Therefore, the authors conclude that women with positive Down syndrome screening results can be reassured that this is unlikely to be due to them having had assisted reproduction. However, none of these observed effects was great enough to warrant routine adjustment of marker levels.

Wald et al. examined the positive rate for Down syndrome screening among 150 IVF pregnancies and in 5 non-IVF pregnancies (controls) matched to each case (Wald et al. 1999). Measured maternal serum markers were AFP, unconjugated oestriol (μE3), free βhCG and total βhCG. Corresponding to the previously mentioned results of Barkai et al. and Ribbert et al., median μE3 levels were 6% lower ($P = 0.003$), median free hCG 9% higher ($P = 0.024$) and median total hCG 14% higher ($P = 0.026$) in IVF pregnancies than in control pregnancies. As Barkai et al. reported, in this study there were also no significant differences in AFP levels between cases and controls. Moreover, free βhCG and inhibin A levels were shown to be similar in cases and controls. The screen-positive rate, that is women with a risk of having a Down syndrome pregnancy of 1 in 300 or higher, was 28% in IVF pregnancies, about twice that in controls (17%). The authors explained high βhCG levels in terms of progesterone remaining high in IVF pregnancies, whereas the reason for low μE3 levels remains unclear. Wald et al. advise that, in Down syndrome screening in IVF pregnancies, βhCG and μE3 values should be adjusted to avoid the high screen-positive rate.

Values of βhCG and AFP were also compared between conventional IVF ($n = 46$) conceived pregnancies, oocyte donation conceived pregnancies ($n = 37$), and reference values (Maymon and Shulman 2001). Higher mid-gestation median MOM for βHCG were found in IVF (1.38) and in oocyte donation pregnancies (1.32) than the reference values (0.99). Only oocyte donation pregnancies had elevated AFP levels (1.45 median MOM) (IVF 1.04). The screening results were positive in 11% of IVF and 13% of oocyte donation pregnancies – in no case was a chromosome abnormality detected. On the other hand, the authors claimed that there might be an association with an adverse pregnancy outcome – i.e. gestational diabetes, preeclampsia, oligohydramnion, and small for gestational age infants – in pregnancies with an elevated serum marker level above 1.2 median MOM.

Conclusion

There seems to be no higher rate of chromosome abnormalities with the currently available ART procedures overall. However, with ICSI, a higher rate of gonosomal aberrations in these children cannot be ruled out. Several problems have to be kept in mind, when this problem is analysed. First, up to now no prospective, controlled study has been carried out, in which comparable rates of ICSI and spontaneous pregnancies have been analysed. Until now, the abnormality rates in PND after ICSI have been compared to abnormality rates in spontaneous conceptuses after birth – which might overestimate the rates in ART pregnancies, since a lot of abnormalities will still be lost during the further course up to birth. Second, as with any technique that does not evaluate approximately 100 % of children, there may be an overestimation due to a preselection of diagnosed pregnancies. The problem of gonosomal aberrations, however, has to be communicated to the parents.

Overall, one can see that there is a low acceptance of the advice to perform invasive PND by couples (30–40 %). This can easily be explained by the still increased rate of spontaneous abortions after these procedures. Therefore, an individual indication for each PND has to be established, and the decision also depends on the results of the genetic work-up, which has already been performed in the parents.

Studies show that the rate of invasive diagnosis declines as the technique itself becomes increasingly established. Other, non-invasive, techniques of PND other than prenatal ultrasound have to be critically analysed. Especially problematic is triple testing, since it overestimates the risks in these pregnancies due to the normal values of the serologic markers used: hCG levels seem to be higher as reference values, and in some studies AFP levels have also been found to be increased.

Ultrasound, on the other hand, is an excellent method for identifying pregnancies at risk for abnormalities in the fetuses. A combination of an early ultrasound with NT measurement at the end of the first trimester, and a high resolution ultrasound at the end of the second trimester including echocardiography seems to be the optimal approach – so-called "genetic sonography". However, even with ultrasound, individual counselling has to be done before each diagnosis.

5 Obstetric Outcome of Pregnancies After Assisted Reproduction

Georgine Huber, Michael Ludwig

Besides the health of children born after ART procedures, the health of the mother has to be the focus of research. As already outlined in previous chapters, there might be a comparable risk of spontaneous abortions, but an increased risk of ectopic and especially heterotopic pregnancies. It has been suggested in the literature that the health of pregnant women may be endangered by the numerous risks caused by multiple pregnancies such as pre-eclampsia, gestational diabetes, premature onset of labour, premature rupture of membranes and finally a higher incidence of non-spontaneous deliveries.

Regarding the newborns, several studies have dealt with the high number of problems due to prematurity and low birth weight, which may increase the perinatal morbidity and mortality in the children. Moreover, it has been hypothesized that each of the different therapies may carry risks for the developing embryo and its genetic health: previous hormonal treatment of the mother and its potential teratogenic effects, potential mechanical damage to the oocyte during retrieval, the use of potentially teratogenic substances in culture mediums or the passing on of genetic defects responsible for sperm impairment.

In the early days of ART in the late 1970s and early 1980s aspects of treatment protocols, patient characteristics and their effect on the success rate were studied extensively. During recent years, the possible risks, adverse effects and the course of subsequent pregnancies have become of wider interest. An overview of the literature and published research data concerning the obstetric outcome of pregnancies after assisted reproduction is presented below.

Singletons Conceived by ART
Versus Spontaneously Conceived Pregnancies

The incidence of preterm deliveries and of low birth weight is higher in pregnancies resulting from ART than from spontaneous conception. This may be mainly due to the higher rate of multiple births after assisted reproduction. However, some have proposed that singleton pregnancies also carry a higher risk of obstetric complications. This suggests that several factors are likely to contribute to a greater risk of obstetric complications in ART than in natural pregnancies: the women tend to be older when getting pregnant and may have a medical history of tubal or uterine disease or endocrine problems, which may increase the background risk for these pregnancies (Lancaster 1985). According to an overview of the literature on children after IVF by Buitendijk, most of the studies into outcomes of IVF singleton pregnancies have shortcomings as to the control groups or the number of control factors, but still there is evidence that IVF singleton pregnancies show a worse outcome than spontaneously conceived singleton pregnancies (Buitendijk 1999).

In a case-control study, Maman et al. compared 169 singleton pregnancies achieved by IVF and 646 singleton pregnancies achieved by ovulation induction with two control groups ($n = 469$ and $n = 1902$) of spontaneously conceived pregnancies (Maman et al. 1998). The groups were matched in terms of maternal age, gestational age and parity. The IVF group had a significantly higher rate of non-insulin-dependent gestational diabetes mellitus (21.3% versus 11.3%, $P = 0.002$). The rate in the ovulation induction group was also significantly higher than in its control group (12.7% versus 6.9%, $P < 0.001$). The rate of pregnancy-induced hypertension was higher in the IVF and ovulation induction groups (9.5% and 9.3%) than in the control groups (5.2% and 6.2%). This was statistically significant for the ovulation induction group and its control ($P = 0.008$). Significantly more babies in the IVF and ovulation induction groups were delivered by caesarean section (47.3% and 18.4%, $P < 0.001$) than in the spontaneously conceived groups (19.8% and 13.1%, $P = 0.001$). The authors hypothesized that gestational diabetes mellitus and pregnancy-induced hypertension could be related to the relatively high prevalence of polycystic ovary syndrome (PCOS) among patients undergoing IVF and ovulation induction. The high rate of caesarean sections in the groups of IVF and ovulation stimulation might be rooted in the anxiety both of the pregnant woman and her physician to give the best of care for these "precious" pregnancies.

A Dutch matched case-control study by Koudstaal et al. examined the obstetric outcome of 307 IVF pregnancies and 307 spontaneous control pregnancies (Koudstaal et al. 2000a). Matching criteria were maternal age, parity, height, weight, ethnic origin, smoking habit, medical disorders, and obstetric history. Preterm deliveries occurred in 15% of the IVF group and in 5.9% of the control group ($P = 0.005$). The babies of the IVF group were more often small for gestational age (16.2% versus 7.9%, $P < 0.001$). No differences were found in the occurrence of gestational diabetes, pregnancy-induced hypertension, premature rupture of membranes or the rate of spontaneous vaginal deliveries.

Tan et al. compared 763 pregnancies following IVF with a matched control group (Tan et al. 1992). Matching was done for maternal age and multiplicity of the pregnancy. A significantly increased incidence of intrauterine growth retardation ($P < 0.05$) and preterm delivery ($P < 0.001$) was found in singleton IVF pregnancies.

Reubinoff et al. compared 260 singleton IVF pregnancies with 260 naturally conceived singleton pregnancies in a matched case-control study (Reubinoff et al. 1997). The women were matched for maternal age, parity, ethnic origin, location and date of delivery. In contradiction to the studies mentioned above, the IVF pregnancies carried no increased risk as to prematurity, low birth weight, or maternal or fetal complications. The rate of caesarean sections, however, was significantly higher in the group of IVF patients (41.9% versus 15.5%, $P = 0.000001$).

Another matched case-control study included 101 pregnancies conceived by IVF with 101 spontaneous pregnancies (Tallo et al. 1995). Matching was done for maternal age, race, insurance type, neonatal gender, order of gestation and delivery, and date of delivery. It was shown that women with assisted reproduction pregnancies suffered significantly more often from pregnancy-induced hypertension (21% versus 4%, $P = 0.0002$), had significantly more premature labour (44% versus 22%, $P = 0.001$), needed significantly more labour induction (25% versus 1%, $P = 0.0001$) and had significantly more preterm deliveries (37% versus 21%, $P = 0.009$) than their controls. However, the authors claim that the number of multiple gestations in this study (72 twins and 9 triplets) accounted for most of the complications.

Doyle et al. found similar results as to preterm delivery, low birth weight and small for gestational age singletons resulting from IVF (Doyle et al. 1992). Obstetric data from 648 singleton IVF babies born in the UK between 1978 and 1987 were compared with the overall number of spontaneously conceived babies in England and Wales during this period. Of the babies born following IVF, 13% were preterm compared with 6% in England and Wales ($P < 0.001$), 11% were of low birth weight compared with 7% in England and Wales ($P < 0.001$) and 17% were defined as small for gestational age compared with 10% of spontaneously conceived singletons ($P < 0.01$). Maternal age did not emerge as a risk factor for prematurity, low birth weight or small for gestational age in this study. The authors suggest that other factors such as the cause of infertility influence obstetric outcome. Women with tubal obstruction had a lower risk of adverse perinatal outcome than couples with idiopathic or male infertility: low birth weight occurred in 9.1% of babies with mothers having tubal obstruction versus 17.2% with parents having idiopathic or male infertility ($P = 0.01$).

In a retrospective Swedish cohort study Bergh et al. compared 5,856 babies born following IVF with all babies born in the general population ($n = 1,505,724$) between 1982 and 1995. Preterm births occurred in 30.3% of all IVF deliveries compared with 6.3% in the general population, low birth weight in 27.4% compared with 4.6%, and multiple births in 27% compared with 1% (Bergh et al. 1999). The authors demonstrate that the striking increase in multiple deliveries contains a higher incidence of prematurity, but an increase in prematurity was also seen among singletons conceived by IVF with 11% compared to 5% in the general population.

The results of a case-control study by D'Souza et al. comparing 150 singleton pregnancies conceived by IVF with 278 spontaneously conceived controls (D'Souza et al. 1997) are in agreement with previous findings. The IVF group had a significantly lower mean gestational age (38.4 ± 2.51 versus 39.5 ± 1.25 weeks, $P < 0.00001$), a significantly lower birth weight (3016 ± 641 g, versus 3400 ± 428 g, p < 0.000001) and significantly fewer vaginal deliveries (73.3% versus 93.2%, $P < 0.0001$). A significantly lower birth weight in IVF singletons compared to spontaneously conceived controls was confirmed by the findings of Petersen et al. ($P < 0.025$) in a prospective non-matched series (Petersen et al.

Table 5.1. Singletons conceived by ART versus spontaneously conceived pregnancies. Problems in pregnancies and adverse pregnancy outcomes (*ART* assisted reproduction techniques, *NIDGDM* non-insulin-dependent gestational diabetes mellitus, *PIH* pregnancy-induced hypertension, *SGA* small for gestational age, *LBW* low birth weight, *n.s.* not significant, *n.a.* not available)

Study	No. of ART pregnancies	No. of control pregnancies	NIDGDM (%)		PIH (%)		Caesarean section (%)		Prematurity (%)		SGA (%)		LBW (%)	
			ART	Control	ART	Control	ART	Control	ART	Control	ART	Control	ART	Control
Maman et al. 1998	169	469	21.3*	11.3*	9.5	5.2	47.3*	19.8*	n.a.		n.s.		n.a.	
Koudstaal et al. 2000a	307	307	n.s.		n.s.		n.s.		15*	5.9*	16.2*	8*	n.a.	
Tan et al. 1992	763	978	n.a.		14*	7.4*	47*	24*	14*	8*	13*	9*	14*	7*
Reubinoff et al. 1997	260	260	n.a.		n.s.		41.9*	15.5*	n.s.		n.s.		n.s.	
Tallo et al. 1995	101	101	n.s.		21*	4*	n.s.		37*	21*	n.a.		42*	27*
Doyle et al. 1992	648	Overall births 1978–1987	n.a.		n.a.		n.a.		13*	6*	17*	10*	11*	7*
Bergh et al. 1999	5856	Overall births 1982–1995	n.a.		n.a.		n.a.		11*	5*	n.a.		9*	3.6*
Dhont et al. 1999	311	311	n.a.		n.a.		n.a.		n.s.		n.a.		n.s.	
D'Souza et al. 1997	150	278	n.a.		n.a.		26.8*	6.8*	12.7*	0.0*	n.a.		14.7*	0.7*
Beck et al. 2001	406	338,737	4.0*	0.8*	6.3*	2.1*	35.7*	19.9*	20.3*	6.7*	n.a.		16.8*	8.0*

* $P < 0.05$.

1995). On the other hand in multiple gestations (16 twins and 4 triplets), similar birth weights were found in the IVF and the control groups.

Dhont et al. found no significant differences between 311 singleton IVF pregnancies and their matched spontaneous pregnancy controls in gestational age, birth weight and incidence of perinatal mortality (Dhont et al. 1999). Matching was done for maternal age, parity, singleton or twin pregnancy and date of delivery. ART twin pregnancies ($n = 115$), however, showed a higher incidence of preterm deliveries than control twin pregnancies (52% versus 42%, $P < 0.05$).

Beck et al. retrospectively compared 406 pregnancies conceived after IVF with 338,737 spontaneously conceived pregnancies as to obstetric complications (Beck et al. 2001). Matching was done for number of fetuses, age and parity. A higher rate of bleeding was found in early pregnancy after IVF (15.7% versus 2.5%, $P < 0.05$), as well as a higher rate of hypertension (6.3% versus 2.1%, $P < 0.05$), gestational diabetes (4.0% versus 0.8%, $P < 0.05$), premature labour (25.7% versus 7.3%, $P < 0.05$) and in consequence a higher rate of prematurity (20.3% versus 6.7%, $P < 0.05$) and caesarean sections (35.7% versus 19.9%, $P < 0.05$).

A summary of all these data is presented in Table 5.1.

According to the findings of most of the studies mentioned above it seems that singleton pregnancies conceived by ART do indeed carry a higher risk of obstetric complications such as prematurity and low birth weight compared to spontaneously conceived pregnancies. It is unclear whether this is related to the ART procedure as such or to other factors such as the infertility itself.

A large cohort study from the US was able to clarify this problem further (Schieve et al. 2002). In this study, 42,463 children born after ART in the years 1996 and 1997 were compared with 3,389,098 children born in 1997. In the study cohort, 43% of children were singletons, 43% were twins, 12% were triplets and 1% were quadruplets or higher order multiples. When only the 16,730 singletons in the study group after adjustment for mother's age were analysed, there was a significantly increased risk for low (odds ratio 1.8, 95% CI 1.7–1.8) and very low birth weight (odds ratio 1.7, 95% CI 1.5–1.9). Interestingly, this risk disappeared, when 180 children from pregnancies with a gestational carrier, i.e. surrogate motherhood, were analysed (odds ratio 1.2, 95% CI 0.6–1.8). Of course, the number of children in the second analysis was much smaller. However, this clearly shows that the influence of the mother on the outcome was substantial: even without additional risk factors, infertility per se contributed to the problem of low birth weight children.

Singleton Versus Multiple Pregnancies After IVF or IVF/ICSI

The Australian In Vitro Collaboration Group studied the outcome of 138 pregnancies resulting from IVF between the years 1980 and 1983 (Australian In Vitro Fertilisation Collaborative Group 1985). Of the singletons, 19% were delivered before term. This proportion is more than three times higher than the comparable proportion in the general Australian population at that time, which was used as a control group (6.2%). Multiple births, occurring in 22% of the total births – compared to 1% in the Australian population – were another major factor for prematurity. All four triplet births, which were included in this analysis, and 23% of the twin births occurred before 37 weeks of gestation.

In accordance with these findings, 19% of the singletons after IVF had a birth weight less than 2500 g; in twins the rate was 42% and in triplets 82%. However, this study involved population figures as controls, and it is unclear whether adjustment for factors such as maternal age and parity was done.

In a retrospective study, Wennerholm et al. found a multiple birth rate of 27% in a group of 100 pregnancies achieved by IVF-ET (Wennerholm et al. 1991). Hypertension, preterm labour and premature rupture of membranes occurred in 22% of these pregnancies. Of the singleton pregnancies, 11% were complicated by hypertension, 18% by preterm labour and 10% by premature rupture of membranes. While 20% of singletons were born before term and 16% had a birth weight less than 2500 g, the rate of prematurity was 56% for multiples and 57% of these babies weighed less than 2500 g.

Govaerts et al. retrospectively compared 145 singleton and 145 multifetal (twins and triplets) matched pregnancies conceived after IVF and ICSI (Govaerts et al. 1998). The rate of multiple gestations was similar in both groups – 31% in IVF and 35% in ICSI. For singletons there was no difference in obstetric complications, prematurity, birth weight or gestational age at the time of delivery between IVF and ICSI. Twins conceived from ICSI were delivered 1 week later than those from IVF, and thus the birth weight of these twins was significantly higher (2488 ± 507 g versus 2281 ± 561 g, $P < 0.05$). Accordingly, more prenatal hospitalizations for risk of preterm labour or rupture of membranes were found in IVF twin pregnancies compared to ICSI pregnancies (44.4% versus 23.5%). The number of caesarean sections was twice as frequent for twins (41% and 33%) versus singletons (21% and 17%) in ICSI and IVF pregnancies, respectively.

A summary of these data is presented in Table 5.2.

Confirming the studies discussed above, Wennerholm and Bergh (2000), found a prematurity rate of 8.4%, 42.3%, and 100% in singleton, twin, and triplet pregnancies after IVF (Wennerholm and Bergh 2000). There was, however, no difference in obstetric outcome between IVF and ICSI pregnancies, nor did the severity of male subfertility influence the outcome.

Strömberg et al. showed in a register-based study from Sweden that the risk of neurological sequelae in children born after IVF was 1.4 times higher than in spontaneously conceived children (Strömberg et al. 2002). However, after performing a logistic regression analysis, gestational age and birth weight had a significant influence on the risk of neurological problems, but a history of IVF did not. Further analysis led to the conclusion that it was the high number of multiple births, and not the ART procedure, that increased the risk for newborns. Finally, another group from Sweden showed that it is mainly the rate of multiple pregnancies that contributes to a higher number of hospital stays in children born after IVF (Ericson et al. 2002).

Table 5.2. Singleton versus multiple pregnancies after ART. Problems in pregnancies and adverse pregnancy outcomes (*ART* Assisted reproduction techniques, *LBW* low birth weight, *PROM* premature rupture of membranes, *PIH* pregnancy-induced hypertension, *n.a.* data not available)

Study	No. of ART pregnancies	No. of control pregnancies	Singleton/multiple (%) ART	Control	Prematurity, singleton/multiple (%) ART	Control	LBW, singleton/multiple (%) ART	Control	PIH, singleton/multiple (%) ART	Control	Preterm labour, singleton/multiple (%) ART	Control	PROM, singleton/multiple (%) ART	Control	Caesarean section, singleton/multiple (%) ART	Control
Australian IVF 1985	138	Overall births 1980–1983	78/22*	99/1*	19*/23	6.2*/n.a.	19/42	n.a.	n.a.		n.a.		n.a.		n.a.	
Wennerholm et al. 1991	100	n.a.	73/27		20/56		16/57		11/22		18/22		10/22		n.a.	
Govaerts et al. 1998 IVF	145		69/31		n.a.		4.8/ 51.8*		7.6/ 11.1*		12.1/ 44.4*				17/33*	
ICSI	145		65/35				3.2/ 47.1*		9.0/ 26.5*		9.0/ 26.5*				21/41*	

* Statistically significant.

All these data therefore underline the necessity to reduce the number of multiple pregnancies as much as possible in order to guarantee the best possible outcome for the children born.

Multiple Pregnancies After ART
Versus Spontaneously Conceived Multiple Pregnancies

Since previous chapters have shown that it is not only mainly the problem of infertility itself – which cannot be changed – but also the risk of multiple pregnancies that contributes to the worse outcome of ART pregnancies, the question arises as to whether multiple pregnancies after ART do worse than those after spontaneous conception.

A multiple pregnancy rate of 25% to 30% for IVF is reported in the literature (Buitendijk 1999). The ESHRE ICSI Task Force Report presents similar figures for ICSI procedures (Tarlatzis and Bili 1998).

One study compared 105 twin pregnancies resulting from IVF with 297 spontaneously conceived twin pregnancies (Bernasko et al. 1997). After controlling for maternal age and parity, a significantly higher incidence of low birth weight (72% versus 59%) and discordant birth weight (23% versus 14%) was found in IVF twin pregnancies. Discordant fetal growth mainly occurs in monochorionic pregnancies. Therefore it is surprising to see the higher rate of discordance in the IVF group, since IVF pregnancies are in most cases dizygotic. However, a decreased functioning of the placenta might explain the higher rate of discordant birth weight and of low birth weight in the IVF group. There was no difference in prematurity rates between the two groups.

A further Dutch study also looked for differences in the outcome of twin IVF as compared to spontaneously conceived twin pregnancies from the same hospital – selected according to different matching parameters (maternal age, parity, ethnic origin, date of parturition, smoking habits, and body height and weight) (Koudstaal et al. 2000b). In each group, 96 pregnancies were recruited resulting in the birth of 192 children. Maternal characteristics were comparable, or even in favour of IVF children, since monozygosity was higher in the spontaneously conceived group (23.3% versus 2.3%). The mode of delivery and gestational age at birth were comparable. The incidence of low birth weight (60.8% versus 44.4%, $P = 0.02$) and discordant birth weight of more than 25% difference (22.9% versus 11.5%, $P = 0.04$), however, were significantly higher in twins born after IVF as compared to those born after spontaneous conception (Koudstaal et al. 2000b).

Friedler et al. studied 56 triplet pregnancies conceived after unspecified ART, comparing them with 82 triplet pregnancies after ovulation induction (gonadotropin stimulation, clomiphene citrate) and 13 triplet pregnancies conceived spontaneously (Friedler et al. 1994). The mean gestational age of the triplets following ART was not different from those conceived by ovulation induction but was significantly shorter than in the pregnancies conceived spontaneously (33.2 versus 35.3 weeks). Triplets resulting from ART had a significantly lower mean birth weight than children following spontaneous conception (1743 versus

1963 g). No difference was found in low birth weight rate between the groups, although the rate of very low birth weight (< 1500 g) after ART and ovulation induction was significantly different from spontaneously conceived triplets (31%, 30% and 10%, respectively). This study did not control for maternal characteristics, so no conclusion can be drawn as to whether maternal features may have influenced the worse outcome in the group of ART and ovulation induction compared with the group of spontaneously conceived pregnancies.

In contrast to the results of the study mentioned above, Olivennes et al. (1996), comparing 72 twin pregnancies following IVF, 82 twin pregnancies following ovulation induction and 164 twin pregnancies conceived spontaneously, found no difference in prematurity rates (39%, 45% and 40%), small for gestational age children (18%, 23% and 23%) or perinatal mortality (3%, 3% and 4%) between the three groups, respectively. This study, however, did not control for other maternal characteristics.

A summary of these data is presented in Table 5.3.

Table 5.3. Multiple pregnancies after ART versus spontaneous multiple pregnancies. Pregnancy problems and adverse pregnancy outcomes (*SGA* small for gestational age)

Study	No. of pregnancies	Low birth weight (%)	Very low birth weight (< 1500 g) (%)	Discordant birth weight (%)	Mean gestational age	Prematurity	SGA	Perinatal mortality
Bernasko et al. 1997								
ART	105	72		23				
Spontaneous	297	59*		14*				
Friedler et al. 1994								
ART	56		31		33.2 weeks			
Ovulation	82		30		33.4 weeks			
Spontaneous	13		10*		35.3 weeks*			
Koudstaal et al. 2000								
ART	96			22.9	251 ± 27 days			
Spontaneous	96			11.5	256 ± 26 days			
Olivennes et al. 1996								
IVF	72					39	18	3
Ovulation induction	82					45	23	3
Spontaneous	164					40	23	4

* Statistically significant.

Higher Order Multiple Pregnancies Following ART

A higher order multiple pregnancy is defined as a pregnancy with at least three fetuses. A small retrospective study of 48 multiple pregnancies (36 twins, 8 triplets, 2 quadruplets, 2 quintuplets) after IVF-ET revealed a 55.5% rate of caesarean section with twins. All high-grade multiples were delivered abdominally. Of the mothers of twins, 28.8% had premature labour, 19.4% had premature rupture of membranes, and 5.6% suffered from pregnancy-induced hypertension. Of the mothers of triplets and of quadruplets, 50% had premature labour, and both mothers of quintuplets suffered premature labour. Of the mothers of triplets, 37.5% had premature rupture of membranes, and 25% pregnancy-induced hypertension (Causio et al. 1995).

Similar findings were presented by Ho et al. (1996). In a retrospective study, pregnancy-related complications and pregnancy outcome were investigated in 34 triplet pregnancies resulting from ART. The most common pregnancy problem was preterm labour (56%), followed by premature rupture of membranes (35%), pregnancy-induced hypertension (15%), cervical incompetence (12%) and abruptio placentae (12%). There was a caesarean section rate of 79.4% versus 20.6% vaginal deliveries. All seven neonates with asphyxia occurred in the vaginal delivery group, and three of them had severe asphyxia with an APGAR score of < 3.

A summary of these data is presented in Table 5.4.

Obstetric Outcome of Pregnancies After Cryopreservation

In IVF treatment superovulation can lead to a high number of oocytes to be fertilized. If too many embryos are thus created, surplus embryos can be frozen in order to be thawed in subsequent cycles. However, cryopreservation and thawing may involve major cellular changes and it is a matter of discussion as to whether these procedures have adverse effects for the children born from this

Table 5.4. Higher order multiple pregnancies following ART. Complications in pregnancies and adverse pregnancy outcomes (*PROM* premature rupture of membranes, *PIH* pregnancy-induced hypertension, *n.a.* data not available from the study)

Study	No. of higher grade pregnancies	Caesarean section (%)	Preterm labour (%)	PROM (%)	PIH (%)	Cervical incompetence (%)	Abruptio placentae haemorrhage (%)
Causio et al. 1995	36 twins	55.5	28.8	19.4	5.6	n.a.	n.a.
	8 triplets	100	50	37.5	25	n.a.	n.a.
	2 quadruplets	100	50	n.a.	n.a.	n.a.	n.a.
	2 quintuplets	100	100	n.a.	50	n.a.	n.a.
Ho et al. 1996	34 triplets	79.4	56	35	15	12	12

technique. So far the number of studies concerning the effects of cryopreservation on human embryos is limited. The following text gives an overview of the literature on this topic. For a better understanding of the data, we have subdivided the presentation into non-controlled and controlled studies.

Descriptive Studies Without Control Groups

Frydman et al. describe the obstetric outcome of 28 pregnancies (including three twin pregnancies) resulting from cryopreserved embryos (Frydman et al. 1989). There was no matched control group. Obstetric complications consisted of premature labour in 21.4 %, pregnancy-induced hypertension in 10.3 % and breech presentation at term in 12 %. Premature birth occurred in all twin pregnancies and in 4 % of the singletons. The caesarean section rate in this series was 21.4 %.

Olivennes et al. studied the perinatal outcome of 89 children (75 singletons and 7 twins) conceived from cryopreserved embryos (Olivennes et al. 1996). No control group was employed. Of the singletons and twins, respectively, 14.7 % and 85.7 % were born prematurely, and 8 % of the singletons and 28.6 % of the twins were small for gestational age. The authors conclude that so far there is no evidence from human data that cryopreservation carries risks for the children born, but it must be emphasized that the number of studied children was very small and no control groups were employed.

A summary of these data is presented in Table 5.5.

Controlled Studies

In a retrospective study, Wada et al. compared the birth characteristics and perinatal mortality of babies conceived from cryopreserved embryos with those resulting from IVF and fresh embryo transfer (Wada et al. 1994). In the cryopreservation group a total of 232 babies were born. Of these, 185 were singletons,

Table 5.5. Pregnancy complications in cryopreserved pregnancies. Descriptive studies without control groups (*PIH* pregnancy-induced hypertension, *SGA* small for gestational age)

Study	No. of cryopreserved pregnancies	Pregnancy complications (%)
Frydman et al. 1989	28 (25 singletons, 3 twins)	Premature labour (all): 21.4 PIH (all): 10.3 Breech position (all): 12.0 Premature birth: singletons 4, twins 100
Olivennes et al. 1996	89 (75 singletons, 7 twins)	Premature birth: singletons 14.7, twins 85.7 SGA: singletons 8, twins 28.6

43 were twins, and 4 were triplets. In the fresh IVF-ET group a total of 763 infants were born. Of these, 592 were singletons, 144 were twins, and 27 were triplets. There was no difference in the incidence of twin or triplet births or in the mean gestational age at birth between the two groups. Fewer cryopreserved twins than IVF-ET twins were delivered preterm (33 versus 58%, $P < 0.05$) and fewer cryopreserved twins than IVF-ET twins had a low birth weight (38 versus 53%, $P < 0.05$). Major congenital malformations were observed in two (1%) of the cryopreservation group babies, which was significantly fewer than the 32 infants seen in the IVF-ET group (3%, $P < 0.05$).

Wennerholm et al. evaluated the obstetric and perinatal outcome of 270 children resulting from 163 singleton, 49 twin, and 3 triplet pregnancies conceived from transfer of cryopreserved embryos (Wennerholm et al. 1997). The two control groups consisted of 209 children born after IVF-ET and 209 spontaneously conceived children. The controls were matched according to maternal age, parity, plurality and date of delivery. The total numbers of hypertensive complications in pregnancy were similar in the three groups (7.2%, 7.7% and 6.2% in pregnancies following cryopreservation, IVF and spontaneous conception). Premature rupture of membranes occurred significantly more often in the ART groups than in the spontaneous pregnancy group (cryopreservation versus spontaneous pregnancy group, $P = 0.037$; IVF-ET versus spontaneous pregnancy group, $P = 0.019$). No difference was found in the mean gestational age. The mean birth weights for singletons were comparable in all groups. Twins conceived from IVF-ET had a significantly lower birth weight than spontaneously conceived twins (2441 ± 666 versus 2673 ± 647 g, $P = 0.014$). The highest frequency of caesarean sections was found in the cryopreserved singleton group, and this was significantly higher than in the spontaneously conceived group (26.3% versus 16.3%, $P = 0.038$). The incidence of malformations showed no difference between the three groups.

Aytoz et al. compared the obstetric outcome of 153 IVF and 94 ICSI pregnancies obtained after the transfer of cryopreserved embryos with 181 IVF and 128 ICSI pregnancies obtained after fresh embryo transfer as controls (Aytoz et al. 1999). The controls were matched according to maternal age, parity and the date of embryo transfer. Pregnancy outcome for singletons and twins was compared separately. There were 126 singletons (82.4%) and 27 twins (17.6%) in the cryopreservation group and 134 singletons (68.5%) and 56 twins (30.9%) in the fresh IVF group. The multiple pregnancy rate was significantly higher in the fresh IVF group ($P < 0.01$). In the cryopreservation ICSI group, 79 singletons (84.0%) and 15 twins (16.0%) were born, and in the fresh ICSI group, 88 singletons (68.8%) and 40 twins (31.3%) were born. Again the multiple pregnancy rate was significantly higher in the fresh ICSI group ($P < 0.05$). No significant difference was found between the groups as to mean gestational age at birth and mean birth weights. However, the frequencies of infants with low birth weight in the frozen IVF group (16.1%) and ICSI group (12.1%) were significantly lower than those in the fresh IVF group (32.2%) and ICSI group (32.7%) ($P < 0.001$). The major malformation rates were not different within the four groups.

A summary of these data is presented in Table 5.6.

Table 5.6. Pregnancy complications in cryopreserved pregnancies. Controlled studies (*PIH* pregnancy-induced hypertension, *PROM* premature rupture of membrane, *n.a.* not available, *n.d.* no difference)

Study	No. of cryopreserved pregnancies	No. of control pregnancies	Incidence of multiples (%)		Prematurity (%)		Low birth weight (%)		PIH (%)		PROM (%)	
			Cryopreserved	Control	Cryopreserved	Control	Cryopreserved	Control	Cryopreserved	Control	Cryopreserved	Control
Wada et al. 1994	323	763	n.d.		33*	58*	38*	53*	n.a.		n.a.	
Wennerholm et al. 1997	270	209 IVF	n.a.		n.a.		n.a.		7.2	7.7	8.6*	9.1*
		209 spontaneous								6.2		3.3*
Aytoz et al. 1999												
IVF	153	181	17.6*	30.9*	n.a.		16.1*	32.2*	n.a.		n.a.	
ICSI	94	128	16.0*	31.3*			12.1*	32.7*				

* Statistically significant.

Conclusion

Overall, the higher rate of multiple pregnancies following each ART technique is a critical factor. It increases the risk for the children born after ART severalfold. For IVF, however, there is also a higher risk for singletons. These pregnancies show a higher risk of premature birth, premature rupture of membranes and lower birth weight. On the other hand, the mothers have a higher risk of pregnancy complications such as pre-eclampsia. Different studies have shown that these risks do not exist in a direct comparison with ICSI pregnancies. The risks also disappear when a surrogate mother, rather than the infertile mother, carries the pregnancy.

Therefore, it seems that certain types of infertility per se do contribute to the risk of pregnancy complications – but not the ART procedure used to induce the pregnancy. This has to be included in the counselling of these patients.

Regarding pregnancies following cryopreservation, there is no increased risk as compared to those established following transfer of fresh non-frozen embryos.

6 Oocyte Donation

Anna Sophie Seelig, Michael Ludwig

Introduction

Besides the possibility of ART in the homologous system, techniques which use a heterologous system have become increasingly used. Advances in ART have attempted to address the problem of declining fecundity due to poor ovarian reserve by using the technique of oocyte donation, i.e. using an oocyte from another woman to achieve fertilization and subsequent pregnancy. The first pregnancy derived from oocyte donation resulted in miscarriage (Trounson et al. 1983), but a successful pregnancy in a 25-year-old woman with premature ovarian failure was reported only 1 year later by the same group (Lutjen et al. 1984)

Since the introduction of oocyte donation, a great increase in the number of families benefiting from oocyte donation continues to be recorded. According to the Society for Assisted Reproductive Technology (SART), 5237 oocyte donation cycles were performed in the United States in 1998 with an overall delivery rate of 41.2% per transfer (SART 2002). This great demand for oocyte donation seems to be due to social and biological life changes. Women tend to postpone childbearing for reasons which may include, among others: the priority to establish a career, the availability of reliable methods of birth control, the rising incidence of divorce and a wish for children with the new partner, and the increase in mean life expectancy that has occurred over the last 100 years. Biological factors that reflect waning oocyte quality of women of advanced age include a greater incidence of luteal phase deficiency, an increased incidence of embryonic chromosomal abnormalities and subsequent spontaneous abortion. Other factors influencing fertility include an increasing chance of exposure to sexually transmitted diseases and resultant pelvic inflammatory disease, and an alteration of normal pelvic anatomy due to the development of uterine leiomyomas and endometriosis.

Since oocyte donation is a well-established method of assisted reproduction most women who were formerly classified as infertile can now become pregnant and give birth. However, a general concern has been raised over possible risks of oocyte donation for the health of both the women and the fetus as well as the newborn child, which may be other than those known for ART procedures in the homologous system.

Here we present information on the clinical aspects of oocyte donation. Our main interest lies in the obstetric course and outcome of these cycles. However, since oocyte donation is quite different from most other ART, aspects of donor motivation, anonymity versus non-anonymity, and the handling by donors of the donation process in the future must also be discussed, since this might have an influence on family structures and development of the children.

Oocyte Recipients and Donors

Potential oocyte recipients can be classified into two distinct groups: those with and those without ovarian function. The first group consists of women at risk of transmitting genetic diseases and women with repetitive failures after IVF or the development of only a few follicles, resulting in poor oocyte recovery (Rosenwaks 1987; Cornet et al. 1990; Van Steirteghem et al. 1992). The second group includes women with premature menopause, surgically absent ovaries, ovarian failure induced by chemotherapy and/or radiotherapy and gonadal dysgenesis with or without chromosomal aberrations (Pados et al. 1992). Furthermore, women who are peri- or postmenopausal and who still want to get pregnant also have to be included in this group (Antinori et al. 1993).

Hormonal Substitution for Oocyte Recipients

Depending on whether the recipient retains ovarian function or has ovarian failure, the endometrial preparation for the embryo transfer follows two distinct directions.

In patients with retained ovarian function, appropriate synchronization between donor and recipient must be obtained since the window of implantation is rather limited (Rosenwaks 1987). Luteinizing hormone (LH) determination in both donor and recipient cycles has been used in order to avoid uteroembryonic asynchrony (Rogers et al. 1988). Administration of a gonadotropin-releasing hormone agonist (GnRH-a) in the donor and recipient cycles or cryopreservation of donated embryos (Van Steirteghem et al. 1987; Pados et al. 1992) can be used to circumvent the problem of synchronization (Cameron et al. 1989; Serhal 1990).

Patients with ovarian failure require adequate hormonal substitution to produce endometrial growth and differentiation. Routinely, exogenous oestrogen and progesterone are administered in various concentrations and application forms in order to mimic the cyclic fluctuations of ovarian hormones in the normal cycle. The effectiveness of steroid replacement therapy has been assessed in preparatory cycles by serial determination of oestrogen and progesterone concentrations and by endometrial biopsies on day 21 (Noyes et al. 1950; Bourgain et al. 1990).

Oestrogen replacement can be administered orally, transdermally or in the form of transvaginal rings. Orally administered oestrogens are exposed to the intestinal milieu where the bioavailability of the circulating oestrogens is reduced by 30%. Transdermal administration is therefore preferred by most IVF centres.

Progesterone replacement therapy can be delivered in the form of oral tablets, intravaginal suppositories, tablets or cream and intramuscular (i.m.) injection. The most reliable progesterone concentrations can be achieved via the vaginal or i.m. route, since oral administration of progesterone results in a low bioavailability (< 10%) because progesterone is metabolized in the liver. Furthermore, many nonphysiological metabolites are created, which result in a high rate of side effects (Devroey and Pados 1998).

Oocyte Donors

The number of women requesting oocyte donation is far greater than the availability of women willing to participate as oocyte donors. Donor recruitment is a difficult endeavour. The known time, effort, commitment, discomfort, and minor risks derived from ovarian stimulation and oocyte retrieval continue to limit donor availability (Ahuja et al. 1997; Englert and Govaerts 1998a). Furthermore, a considerable number of potential donors may have a positive finding on medical, genetic, or psychological testing that prohibits donation. In the view of different international organizations, such as the ASRM, or groups which actively work in this field, donors should be screened for hepatitis B and C, and HIV. Drug and alcohol problems or active smoking should be excluded. Moreover, donors should undergo a psychological evaluation and should be assessed for genetic factors (Devroey et al. 1989). In addition, each candidate should be matched to the potential recipient on physical characteristics (e.g. blood type, ethnicity, height, weight and colouring) (Schover et al. 1991). Donors need to understand the boundaries of their role and need to be fully capable and free from any kind of coercion in giving informed consent (Baetens et al. 2000). Because of the rigorous testing for potential genetic or infectious diseases and because of the extraordinary commitment required, experience has shown that < 50% of the donors starting the process of screening are actually approved to proceed to stimulation and retrieval (Moomjy et al. 2000a).

Some statistics on the recruitment of oocyte donors have been reported (Murray and Golombok 2000). A survey by these authors showed that in 1 year about 6000 potential donors contacted the 55 clinics within this survey, and about 1400 entered the screening process. Of these, about 200 were found to be unsuitable as donors as a result of screening, and about 1100 of the 1200 donors accepted after screening, finally donated oocytes. Therefore, 18% of those who originally plan to donate oocytes finally do so. On the other hand, more than 90% of donors accepted after screening actually donate.

Whether payment influences the motivation of different subgroups of donors is a matter of ongoing debate. Some recent work, however, did not show a difference in major demographic characteristics – independently of whether 2500 USD or 5000 USD was paid for oocyte donation (German et al. 2001).

Oocyte donors can be subdivided into two groups, those who know the recipient and those who are anonymous. The first are mostly friends or relatives. The latter include both patients undergoing IVF who donate their supernumerary oocytes altruistically or for a certain financial compensation (oocyte sharing programmes) and patients who undergo tubal sterilization and agree to ovarian stimulation. It should be noted, however, that the advent of cryo-preservation has decreased substantially the number of oocytes available for donation from IVF patients.

Another concept in the recruitment of oocyte donors, so-called "personalized anonymity", was introduced by a Belgium group (Englert et al. 1996; Englert and Govaerts 1998b). Each recipient couple attends with a donor, but the oocytes from that donor are assigned to another recipient couple, who in return provide the oocytes from their donor to the other couple. This exchange is arranged by the fertility centre in such a manner that the recipient couples have no contact with their donor, and anonymity is guaranteed. In fact, the authors proposed that they have a 100% pregnancy rate per donation when they distribute the oocytes to several recipients – which is a quite important advantage in the light of the low number of available donors.

This is confirmed by others who have performed shared oocyte donation – i.e. sharing oocytes from one donor to two recipients (Moomjy et al. 2000b). This has resulted in the achievement of a clinical pregnancy rate of 109.5% and a delivery rate of 95.4% per oocyte donor – in a programme with a mean recipient age of 40.9 ± 4.4 years. This is, however, only possible if more than eight oocytes per donor are retrieved, leading to a mean of 8.3 oocytes per recipient.

Follow-up of Oocyte Donors

Several donor follow-up studies have been reported (Schover et al. 1991; Rosenberg and Epstein 1995; Fielding et al. 1998; Ahuja et al. 1998; Kalfoglou and Gittelsohn 2000a).

Most anonymous donors were moderately to extremely satisfied with the donation (Schover et al. 1991; Rosenberg and Epstein 1995) and most former donors were prepared to donate again (Schover et al. 1991; Rosenberg and Epstein 1995; Fielding et al. 1998). Medically most donors did not experience any significant negative effects. In the first follow-up study undertaken by Schover et al. the physical process was mildly negatively tolerated by one-quarter to one-third of the participants (Schover et al. 1991). Rosenberg and Epstein reported that donors had significant discomfort from bloating before and after the retrieval, but the actual retrieval and hormonal injections were well tolerated except for some anxiety relating to self-injecting (Rosenberg and Epstein 1995).

In a follow-up survey of former IVF patients who had donated oocytes to other patients in an egg-sharing programme, donors were typically motivated by empathy for other infertile couples as well as the treatment discount (Ahuja et al. 1998). Even patients who did not become pregnant still supported the idea of egg sharing. Patients rejected the idea that children created from their oocytes were their children.

In a later study, it was found that none of the former donors from IVF clinics, a matching agency, the internet, advertisements, and word of mouth, regretted their decision to donate (Kalfoglou and Gittelsohn 2000a). However, they were not always completely satisfied with the donation experience. The physical process, compensation, quality of medical care, and level of involvement in the process were the primary factors that affected satisfaction.

Concern has been expressed that being a donor or surrogate as a way of coping with a past loss could be counterproductive (Klyman 1986). In the sample of Schover et al., 27% of the donors rated 'making up for a past loss' as a positive aspect of the oocyte donation programme (Schover et al. 1991). The donors who had actually experienced a loss, such as abortion, miscarriage, or a limit on reproduction because of partner resistance, were more likely to give positive ratings. Thus, going through the process of helping another woman can be reparative.

Studies have found that oocyte donors want to be more involved than semen donors (Fielding et al. 1998; Schover et al. 1992) and that they have a great desire to know the outcome of the donation (Schover et al. 1991; Rosenberg and Epstein 1995; Fielding et al. 1998; Kalfoglou and Gittelsohn 2000a). Informing the donor may lead to greater psychological harm or greater risk of family conflict or courtroom tragedy (Schover et al. 1991). But others have argued that knowing the outcome does not appear to increase the donor's thoughts about the resulting child (Kalfoglou and Gittelsohn 2000a). Instead, it appears to increase the 'good feeling' donors have about alleviating the suffering of others. Another reason why donors wanted to know the outcome was a better preparation for the future possibility of meeting the child (Kalfoglou and Gittelsohn 2000a). Some donors also wanted to know the gender and birth date of any resulting offspring in order to prevent their own children from inadvertently marrying or reproducing with a genetic half-sibling. Consanguineous relationships may be statistically unlikely, but the fear is great (Kalfoglou and Gittelsohn 2000a).

More research needs to be done to determine the long-term effects of informing the donor about the outcome before a recommendation can be made. Research is also needed to learn more about the effect of having women travel to complete a donation. Internet-based matches and the use of relatives and friends as donors are increasing long-distance arrangements. Additional follow-up should investigate whether there is an impact on the quality of care for donors who travel. Health-care providers participating in long-distance arrangements also need to consider who is ultimately responsible for the woman's care if there are complications – the health-care provider monitoring the cycle or the health-care provider doing the retrieval.

Donor satisfaction is likely to influence participants' willingness to repeat the experience. It will also generally influence potential donors' willingness to participate and society's acceptance of oocyte donation as a permissible assisted reproductive technology. Improved donor satisfaction is likely to improve donor recruitment and retention.

Effects of Anonymity and Secrecy

Several psychological issues have been identified as important in the process of oocyte donation. First, with regard to motivation, different factors may motivate a woman to consider being an oocyte donor. Although this service may be performed for financial gain, frequently an altruistic reason is a primary motive for participating in an oocyte donation programme (Khamsi et al. 1997; Baetens et al. 2000). The majority of donors in a study by Sauer and Paulson reported that their primary motivation for participation was concern for others' fertility (Sauer and Paulson 1992).

A very controversial issue concerns donor anonymity. The choice of whether to use a known donor can be seen as part of the larger decision of whether to inform the potential child or others about the nature of conception. A study by Khamsi et al. suggests that anonymity was the primary concern for both recipients and donors (Khamsi et al. 1997). The majority of the sample agreed that they would not disclose to family, friends or the child either now or in the future. The data suggest a strong trend for privacy and indicate that issues of confidentiality are very important to individuals in an oocyte donation programme.

Raoul-Duval et al. deliberately chose anonymity (Raoul-Duval et al. 1992). They believe that this enables the recipient couple to construct their own parental status and alleviates their debt to a known donor. Anonymity protects the future child from a potentially harmful multiple parent situation (biological mother, care-giving and social mother), which could be a source of conflict. Their clinical data indicate that oocyte recipients perceive their offspring as immediately, fully and permanently theirs. Exchanges between mother and fetus during pregnancy, childbirth and early mother-infant bonding make these oocyte donation children the true offspring. Biology takes over from genetics and emotional ties are based on the privileged period of pregnancy. They also found that denial is particularly strong in cases of oocyte donation. The anonymity policy for oocyte donation not only protects offspring from having to cope with an impossible lineage (e.g. aunt- mother, genetic mother-aunt) but also aids maternal denial of infertility enabling the leap from infertile woman to mother.

Non-anonymous donation is possible in Belgium, in contrast to many other Western European countries such as Denmark, Spain and the United Kingdom, where oocyte donation is permitted by law but only in an anonymous procedure. A Belgium group found in their study that 68.6% of 144 couples chose known donation (Baetens et al. 2000). Motivation for known donation was fear of genetic material of unknown origin, trust in the personality of the donor, genetic link or physical resemblance between the donor and the recipient woman, practical motives, preference of the donor for known donation, genetic background of the child in order to be able to answer the child's questions. Motivation for anonymous donation was the wish to mark explicit boundaries between the two families involved, independence, protection of the donor, minimization of the link between the donor and the child and practical motive.

Weil et al. found that in known donation, donors rarely considered taking a risk, as compared to almost all anonymous donors (Weil et al. 1994). It is understandable that many women are not willing to donate anonymously, because – as opposed to sperm donation – donating oocytes involves invasive medical treatment for the donor, covering ovarian stimulation and the trans-vaginal retrieval of mature oocytes under anaesthesia. Therefore, it is important to allow each couple to make their own choice, taking into account their con-scious and subconscious wishes, individual history and family structure (Weil et al. 1994).

However, the known donor in particular needs to be counselled for the pos-sibility that the donation may not be successful. This preparation should also include clarification that the donors are not responsible for failures, reassurance that a failure is not a reflection of the donor's fertility and that their contribution is still valuable (Kalfoglou and Gittelsohn 2000b).

A perennial concern when using donated gametes in infertility treatment is the effect on the child. Shenfield and Steele found no evidence that either anonymity or the specific secret of gamete donation is harmful to the child (Shenfield and Steele 1997). Others have reported that in known oocyte donation there is a strong trend for privacy and confidentiality (Khamsi et al. 1997). This concern extends to the child as well. Clearly, disclosing to a child that he or she was conceived as the result of oocyte donation could have quite different im-plications if the donor were known versus anonymous.

Couples who decided not to tell the child were significantly more secretive towards the social environment, while couples who intended to tell the child tended to be significantly more open towards family and friends. Women who had already given birth to a child tended to be significantly more secretive towards the social environment and towards the child, ensuring in this way that the child would not be treated differently by family and friends (Baetens et al. 2000). Follow-up research as regards 'the best interests of the child' is essential. For the time being, all professionals involved in an oocyte donation programme should not convince prospective parents of either openness or anonymity, but should listen to their concerns.

Obstetric Outcome in Oocyte Donation Pregnancies

Women undergoing oocyte donation have a high likelihood of pregnancy suc-cess. In a retrospective study, 418 embryo transfer cycles among 276 recipients of oocyte donation were investigated (Paulson et al. 1997a). The overall clinical pregnancy rate was 36.2% and the cumulative pregnancy rate after four cycles was 87.9%. The overall delivery rate was 29.3% and the cumulative delivery rate after four cycles was 86.1% with no noted decline in per cycle success over con-secutive cycles.

Pregnancies resulting from oocyte donation are unique since they are im-munologically foreign to the recipient. Studying the outcome of these pregnan-cies is important as they may help us to understand the pathophysiology of particular obstetric complications, and to advise oocyte recipients concerning management of their pregnancies.

There are several reported studies on the outcome of pregnancies following oocyte donation (Blanchette 1993; Pados et al. 1994; Sauer et al. 1995; Michalas et al. 1996; Abdalla et al. 1998). Cornet et al. (1990) reported that the obstetric profiles of eight pregnancies after oocyte donation to women with primary ovarian failure were normal. However, this series was quite small, and most other studies indicate that oocyte donation pregnancies should be considered obstetrically as high risk. It is important to determine the factors that affect the outcome of these pregnancies and to identify whether there are any subgroups that could be more at risk in these pregnancies.

Studies have shown that pregnancies after oocyte donation show a high incidence of uterine bleeding, pre-eclampsia, glucose intolerance and gestational diabetes mellitus (GDM), intrauterine growth retardation, preterm labour, and caesarean sections. Indeed, in 1991, a maternal death due to subarachnoid haemorrhage in a twin pregnancy after oocyte donation complicated by hypertension has been reported (Bewley and Wright 1991). However, only a larger series of pregnancies following oocyte donation may help to provide a real estimate of the obstetric risks. Therefore, the characteristics of obstetric complications are presented in Table 6.1. In comparison to patients undergoing traditional IVF, oocyte donation in women of comparable age has obstetric outcomes equal or better (Friedman et al. 1996) (Table 6.2). Indications for caesarean section are listed in Table 6.3. The high caesarean section rate should be attributed, at least partly, to the specific conditions associated with oocyte donation pregnancies. These can include a very advanced maternal age in some studies, and a history of long-standing infertility, pathology of gestation, anxiety of the attending obstetrician about the outcome of the pregnancy and variations throughout the world in the management of such pregnancies.

Perinatal mortality remained at very low levels in all the studies. This undoubtedly reflects the quality of obstetric care, as well as a low incidence of preterm deliveries. As far as maternal mortality is concerned, the studies show no substantial increase. So it can be postulated that pregnancies in these specific groups of patients are not associated with an increased maternal mortality, perhaps as a consequence of the intensive patient preselection on the one hand and intensive obstetric care on the other.

Although oocyte donation pregnancies seem to be at high risk, the majority of the obstetric complications are treatable, and women having oocyte donation should expect an excellent outcome, provided they have good medical care. They should be appropriately counselled about these complications and cared for in centres that can supervise high-risk pregnancies.

The information available regarding the development and health of the children born after oocyte donation is very limited. Raoul-Duval et al. examined a group of 14 infants at the ages of 9 months, 18 months and 3 years (Raoul-Duval et al. 1992, 1994). All the children were born as singletons and all of them showed normal psychomotor and psychological development. In a questionnaire survey by Applegarth et al., 51 offspring aged 12 weeks to 7 years who were born after

Table 6.1. Characteristics of obstetric complications after oocyte donation (*PIH* pregnancy-induced hypertension, *n.a.* not available)

Study clinical	No. of preg-nancies	Uterine bleeding (%)			PIH	Pre-eclampsia (%)	Gesta-tional dia-betes	Intra-uterine growth retarda-tion (%)	Cholest-atic icterus (%)	Placenta previa (%)	Abruptio placenta (%)	Prema-ture labour (%)	Caesarean section (%)	Perinatal mortality (%)	Maternal mortality (%)
		First trim-ester	Second trim-ester	Third trim-ester											
Pados et al. 1994	69	18 (34.6)	1 (1.9)	3 (5.8)	n.a.	17 (32.7)	n.a.	6 (11.5)	2 (3.9)	1 (1.9)	1 (1.9)	1 (1.9)	33 (48)	1.7	0
Abdalla et al. 1998	232	17 (12)	2 (1)	3 (2)	n.a.	10 (7)	n.a.	43 (24.2)	n.a.	n.a.	n.a.	35 (25)	96 (41)	0.57	0
Sauer et al. 1995	17	n.a.	n.a.	n.a.	7	1	2	n.a.	n.a.	n.a.	n.a.	3	n.a.	n.a.	n.a.
Michalas et al. 1996	25[a]	n.a.	n.a.	n.a.	1	0	1	n.a.	n.a.	n.a.	n.a.	5 (20)	n.a.	0	n.a.
	32[b]	n.a.	n.a.	n.a.	3	4	9	n.a.	n.a.	n.a.	n.a.	8 (25)	n.a.	3	n.a.
Blanchette 1993	5	n.a.	n.a.	n.a.	1	1	n.a.	n.a.	n.a.	n.a.	n.a.	2	2 (40)	0	0

[a] < 40 years.
[b] > 40 years.

Table 6.2. Obstetric comparison between oocyte recipients and standard IVF (data according to Friedman et al. 1996)

Parameter	Oocyte donation (%)	Conventional IVF (%)
Multiple gestation	9/22 (40.9)	9/22 (40.9)
Preterm labour	5/22 (22.7)	12/22 (54.6)
Spontaneous vaginal delivery	4/31 (12.9)	11/31 (35.5)
Forceps delivery	13/31 (41.9)	7/31 (22.6)
Caesarean section	14/31 (45.2)	13/31 (41.9)
Placenta previa	2/22 (9.2)	1/22 (4.6)
Birth weight (g)	2924 ± 703	2374 ± 822
Gestational age (weeks)	35 (29–41)	38 (35–42)

Table 6.3. Indications for caesarean section in women with pregnancies following oocyte donation (*n.a.* not available)

	Abdalla et al. 1998	Pados et al. 1994
Malpresentation	16	1
Slow progress in labour	6	1
Fetal distress	10	1
Hypertension	17	5
Multiple pregnancy	10	n.a.
Small stature	1	3
Placenta previa	3	1
Intrauterine growth retardation	4	n.a.
Infertility alone (%)	29 (30)	18 (55)
Wagner disease	n.a.	1
Cholestatic icterus	n.a.	1

oocyte donation were screened (Applegarth et al. 1995). Although a few children experienced health problems at birth, they were all in good health during later stages. Developmental milestones were within normal limits. Söderström-Antilla et al. presented the results of a retrospective study comparing 59 children – 39 singletons and 20 multiples – after oocyte donation with 126 IVF children at the age of 6 months and 4 years (Soderstrom-Anttila et al. 1998). They found no difference concerning the health and well-being between the two groups of oocyte donation children and IVF children, but IVF mothers were more concerned about certain aspects of their child's behaviour than the oocyte donation mothers. Even though the health and socioemotional development of children born after oocyte donation appear to be within the normal range, the psychological long-term consequences of the oocyte donation treatment on the child require further investigation.

The Impact of Age

Fertility rates begin to fall during the fourth decade of life and reach a nadir after the age of 40 years (Maroulis 1991). Moreover, close to 50% of oocytes karyotyped in women over the age of 35 years undergoing IVF are aneuploid (Plachot 1997).

It has been suggested that the age-related decline in human fertility is partly due to a uterine factor (Levran et al. 1991). Uterine blood flow decreases with declining levels of oestradiol, as naturally occurs during the menopause, which may adversely affect the local endometrial environment (de Ziegler et al. 1991). The identification of oestrogen receptors in the wall of the uterine arteries in humans is supportive of this hypothesis (Perrot-Applanat et al. 1988). Fibrotic changes that take place in the walls of the uterine arterial muscle further accent physiological changes that would account for alterations in local blood flow (Crawford et al. 1997). Finally, approximately half of spontaneously aborted pregnancies are chromosomally normal, which implies that a local endomyo-metrial factor may have been responsible for the loss. Whether this is a primary target organ event or secondary to the inability of the ageing corpus luteum to support the pregnancy remains conjectural.

It has been proposed that uterine ageing and low pregnancy rates are due to secretory exhaustion of the uterine epithelium (Edwards 1992). A malfunction of a reduced number of pinopodes in the uterine epithelium could well explain the situation in older women. Furthermore, reactive oxygen species that are pro-duced in the reproductive tract might limit fertility in older women (Edwards 1992). In a study by Cano et al., oocyte recipients older than 40 years had similar implantation rates compared to a group < 40 years of age, but significantly higher abortion rates with a retardation of steroid synthesis were detected (Cano et al. 1995).

However, when correct pharmacological hormone replacement is provided, the endometrium of menopausal women between 40 and 60 years of age demonstrates a normal histological, ultrasonographic, and steroid receptor response (Sauer et al. 1993; Paulson et al. 1997b). As a result, high rates of embryo implantation and pregnancy occur in women of advanced reproductive age undergoing oocyte donation. The rates are higher for recipients of donated oocytes compared to the older population using their own gametes (Sauer et al. 1992). The obstetric outcome of such pregnancies also shows favourable results. The data from studies performed in this area are listed in Tables 6.4 and 6.5.

Nevertheless, oocyte recipients of advanced maternal age seem to have more complicated obstetric courses, with an increased frequency of hypertension, preterm labour requiring tocolysis, pre-eclampsia, glucose intolerance, fetal growth restriction, preterm delivery, placenta previa, and thrombophlebitis (Blanchette 1993; Pados et al. 1994; Borini et al. 1995; Michalas et al. 1996). These studies did not have a control group.

In a study by Wolff et al., 46 patients pregnant following oocyte donation were compared retrospectively with respect to the obstetric outcome with 49 women of similar age who conceived without assistance (Wolff et al. 1997).

Table 6.4. Survey of results with oocyte donation to women of advanced reproductive age or postmenopausal women. Values are means ± SD unless otherwise defined (*n.a.* not available)

Study	Age (years)	No. of recipients	No. of recipient cycles	No. of oocytes per recipient	Fertilization rate (%)	Transfer rate	No. of transfer cycles	No. of embryos transferred per cycle embryo (%)	Implantation rate per transferred (%)	Established pregnancy rate per transfer (%)	Ongoing pregnancy or delivered pregnancy rate per transfer	Ongoing pregnancy rate per transfer (%)	Delivery rate per transfer (%)	Abortion rate (%)
Sauer et al. 1990	>40	7	9	10.8 ±5.8	41	n.a.	8	3.5±1.1	36	6 (75)	62	n.a.	n.a.	n.a
	<40	9	14	13.6 ±6.8	65	n.a.	14	4.8±0.7	27	7 (50)	50	n.a.	n.a.	n.a
	Control group[a]	22	31	5.8 ±3.5	39	n.a.	26	2.6±1.6	7	4 (16)	8	n.a.	n.a.	n.a.
Sauer et al. 1992	>40	65	93	15.2 ±9.0	48.2	n.a.	86	4.4±1.0	19.7	34 (34.5)	33.7	n.a.	n.a.	n.a.
	<40	35	46	15.3 ±6.8	62	n.a.	43	4.7±0.7	15.9	14 (32.6)	30.2	n.a.	n.a.	n.a.
	Control[b] group	57	79	6.7 ±4.1	39.2	n.a.	70	2.9±1.2	4.8	8 (11.4)	8.6	n.a.	n.a.	n.a.
Sauer et al. 1995	>50	36	45	16.2 ±7.5	n.a.	n.a.	45	4.3±1.2	20.6	22 (48.9)	n.a.	n.a.	17 (37.8)	n.a.
Sauer et al. 1996[d]	45–59	162	218	4.5 ±1.1	n.a.	n.a.	212	n.a.	17.4	103 (48.6)	46.8	70 (n.a.)	74 (34.9)	12 (n.a.)

Study	Age													
Antinori et al. 1993	45–63	113		4.13 ±0.62	n.a.	n.a.	n.a.	3.07 ±0.86	12.6	44 (38.9)	n.a.	n.a.	33 (26.5)	8 (18.2)
Borini et al. 1995	> 50	34	61	n.a.	n.a.	n.a.	55	n.a.	18	(32.70)	n.a.	n.a.	n.a.	(5.5)
Yaron et al. 1995	= 45	96	220	n.a.	85.9	n.a.	189	3.5±1.3	n.a.	33 (17.5)	n.a.	7 (n.a.)	19 (57.6)	7 (21.2)
Control group[b]		31	52	n.a.	40.4	n.a.	21	3.6±1.2	n.a.	0	n.a.	0 (0)	0 (0)	0 (0)
Legro et al. 1995	> 42	n.a.	145	7.5±0.4	n.a.	n.a.	n.a.	4.4±0.1	n.a.	n.a.	41 (30.6)	n.a.	n.a.	8 (16.3)
Control group[c]		n.a.	165	7.9±0.4	n.a.	n.a.	n.a.	4.5±0.1	n.a.	n.a.	46 (30.2)	n.a.	n.a.	5 (9.8)

[a] ≥ 40 years with standard IVF.
[b] ≥ 45 years with standard IVF.
[c] ≤ 42 years with oocyte donation.
[d] Results obtained from 1990–1995.

Table 6.5. Perinatal outcome in oocyte donation pregnancies depending on the age of the oocyte recipient. Values are means ± SD unless otherwise defined (*Gest. age* gestational age at delivery in weeks, *n.a.* not available)

Study	Age (years)	Singleton			Twin			Triplet			Quadruplet		Birth weight (g)		
		No.	Gest. age	<37 weeks	No.	Gest. age	<37 weeks	No.	Gest. age	<37 weeks	No.	Gest. age	Singleton	Twin	Triple
Sauer et al. 1992	>40	20	n.a.	n.a.	5	n.a.	n.a.	2	n.a.	n.a.	0	n.a.	n.a.	n.a.	n.a.
	<40	n.a.	n.a.	n.a.	n.a.	n.a.	n.a.	n.a.	n.a.	n.a.	n.a.	n.a.	n.a.	n.a.	n.a.
	Control group[a]	n.a.	n.a.	n.a.	n.a.	n.a.	n.a.	n.a.	n.a.	n.a.	n.a.	n.a.	n.a.	n.a.	n.a.
Sauer et al. 1990	>50	4	n.a.	n.a.	1	n.a.	n.a.	0	n.a.	n.a.	n.a.	n.a.	n.a.	n.a.	n.a.
Pados et al. 1994	23–44	44	n.a.	n.a.	16	n.a.	n.a.	0	n.a	n.a.	0	n.a.	n.a.	n.a.	n.a.
Sauer et al. 1995	50–59	10	38.4 ±1.9	n.a.	6	36.3 ±1.4	n.a.	1	32	n.a.	0	n.a.	3390±715	2352±430	1500/1800/2100
Sauer et al. 1996	45–59	45	38.3 ±1.3	n.a.	24	35.9 ±2.0	n.a.	5	33.5 ±0.7	n.a.	0	n.a.	3218±513	2558±497	1775±190
Antinori et al. 1993	45–63	23	n.a.	n.a.	9	n.a.	n.a.	1	n.a.	n.a.	0	n.a.	n.a.	n.a.	n.a.
Borini et al. 1995	>50	16	n.a.	n.a.	1	n.a.	n.a.	1	n.a.	n.a.	0	n.a.	n.a.	n.a.	n.a.
Yaron et al. 1995	>45	12	n.a.	n.a.	6	n.a.	n.a.	1	n.a.	n.a.	0	n.a.	n.a.	n.a.	n.a.
	Control group[b]	n.a.	n.a.	n.a.	n.a.	n.a.	n.a.	n.a.	n.a.	n.a.	n.a.	n.a.	n.a.	n.a.	n.a.
Legro et al. 1995	>42	28	n.a.	n.a.	11	n.a.	n.a.	1	n.a.	n.a.	1	n.a.	n.a.	n.a.	n.a.
	≤42	27	n.a.	n.a.	14	n.a.	n.a.	5	n.a.	n.a.	0	n.a.	n.a.	n.a.	n.a.
Abdalla et al. 1998	n.a.	105	n.a.	14	32	n.a.	18	3	n.a	3	0	n.a.	n.a.	n.a.	n.a.
Soderstrom-Anttila et al. 1998	>42	39	n.a.	13	n.a.	n.a.	n.a.	n.a.	n.a.	n.a.	n.a.	n.a.	3338±740	n.a.	n.a.
	Control group[c]	68	n.a.	7	n.a.	n.a.	n.a.	n.a.	n.a.	n.a.	n.a.	n.a.	3475±630	n.a.	n.a.

[a] ≥ 40 years with standard IVF. [b] ≥ 45 years with standard IVF. [c] ≤ 42 years with oocyte donation.

Table 6.6. Obstetric outcome in oocyte recipients compared with women of advanced age who conceived without assisted reproductive technologies: all pregnancies (*PROM* premature rupture of membranes, *PIH* pregnancy-induced hypertension) (Wolff et al. 1997)

Outcome	Oocyte recipients (n = 46) (%)	Natural conception (n = 49) (%)
Placenta previa	6.5	2.0
PROM	19.6	4.1
Glucose intolerance of pregnancy	13.0	6.1
PIH	19.6	2.0

Table 6.7. Obstetric outcome in oocyte recipients compared with women of advanced age who conceived without assisted reproductive technologies: singleton pregnancies (*PROM* premature rupture of membranes, *PIH* pregnancy-induced hypertension) (Wolff et al. 1997)

Outcome	Oocyte recipients (n = 23) (%)	Natural conception (n = 48) (%)
Placenta previa	13.0	2.1
PROM	8.7	4.2
Glucose intolerance of pregnancy	13.0	6.3
PIH	13.0	2.1

It has to be noted that in this study half of the oocyte-recipient pregnancies resulted in multiple gestation. When only singleton pregnancies were compared, the obstetric course was similar between the groups. The results of this study are shown in Tables 6.6 and 6.7.

The occurrence of multiple gestations cannot be eliminated in assisted reproductive technologies. Older patients in particular are more inclined to want reduction to singleton gestation. They cite parental demands, financial issues, and their ability to parent in their 60s and 70s as reasons for reduction to singleton gestation (Evans et al. 1997). The concept reinforces the recommendation that the number of embryos transferred should be kept to a minimum to decrease the incidence of multiple gestations, with their inherent perinatal complications. It is the responsibility of the physician to rigorously screen potential recipients before they enter the programme and to follow-up the resulting pregnancies with extreme care.

Conclusion

Using oocyte donation two different populations have to be followed up: one are the oocyte donors, the other the oocyte recipients and their partners. Both seem to do well with this technique. The health risk to the donors seem to be limited, when they are screened before for certain risks. Their motivations have to be critically evaluated. There is still an ongoing debate as to whether the altruistic basis of oocyte donation is the best or not. Facing the great demand for donated oocytes, it is clear, however, that donation on an altruistic basis only will not lead to a sufficient supply of oocytes.

Controlled data regarding the follow-up of pregnancies after oocyte donation are quite rare. Until now, however, it seems to be that there is no increased risk for either the children or the mother after procreation using this very invasive technique. Oocyte donation is also, of course, associated with the risk of multiple pregnancies, which has to be included in the counselling before treatment of these couples. Finally, patients who undergo oocyte donation are a special subgroup of patients with special medical problems and especially with a higher age. These risk factors have to be taken into account in order to estimate the risk on an individual basis and to provide an individual approach to caring for these pregnancies.

7 Congenital Malformations After ART

Annika K. Schröder, Michael Ludwig

As discussed in previous chapters, major concerns about the outcome of IVF pregnancies are related to multiple pregnancies, pregnancy course, and preterm deliveries. But even in the early years of IVF some authors also addressed the possibility that there is an increased risk for congenital malformations (Lancaster 1987). The large number of data now available on this topic help to answer this question more reliably. However, there are problems in the design of almost all the studies. Most studies have included only a limited number of pregnancies and estimations of malformation rates are often uncertain. Other studies are large enough to permit relatively certain estimates of malformation rates, but comparisons have been made with various types of registers while the identification of malformations in children born after IVF are often the result of a detailed follow-up. Some studies include only live-born children, others still-born and live-born children, while other studies also include terminated pregnancies and spontaneous abortions. Furthermore, there is no generally accepted definition of a malformation, often they are divided into minor and major malformations with no clear distinction or without using an internationally accepted malformation classification system. In nearly all studies a major malformation was assumed when either the child was handicapped by the abnormality or if a surgical intervention was necessary. In some studies, no definition of a major malformation was included. An internationally accepted malformation catalogue was used in almost no study. If other definitions of malformations are used in the following review, it is emphasized.

One example of the weaknesses of some studies is the German IVF Registry. This registry in its most recent edition (Deutsches IVF Register 2000) records 29 malformations (1.04%) in 2789 children born after IVF. However, as usual in such registries, neither a definition of malformation nor a standardized procedure for malformation evaluation was included. Furthermore, these data were available only for 86% of all pregnancies. It remains absolutely unclear whether a follow-up regarding malformations was performed at all in most of the pregnancies. On the other hand, this register is the only available means of collecting these data on a large basis, and therefore it is of very high importance.

All these aspects have to be taken into account when comparing malformation rates between the different studies, and when interpreting the study results overall. In the following review, we have tried to differentiate the studies according to the technique used. However, some studies analysed children after conventional IVF as well as after ICSI, and some others mixed up children born after IVF and GIFT. Therefore, in these cases, the data are mentioned only once.

Congenital Malformations After IVF

Lancaster reported the incidence of malformations after IVF from 1981 to 1983 using the Australian data system for congenital malformations and the data system for pregnancies resulting from IVF (Lancaster 1986). These registers included all pregnancies with a gestational age of at least 20 weeks or a birth weight of at least 400 g. Pregnancies terminated after prenatal diagnosis, especially due to chromosomal abnormalities, were sometimes notified as well. Lancaster defined a major congenital malformation to be an anatomical defect or chromosomal abnormality that is present at birth and is either lethal or significantly affects the individual's function or appearance. The incidence of major congenital malformations in the general population obtained from the national congenital malformations data system was 1.5%. After IVF the incidence of major congenital malformations was reported to be 1.1% in 309 pregnancies of at least 20 weeks gestation. In 1987 Lancaster reported 1694 live births and stillbirths of at least 20 weeks gestation and three terminations of pregnancy after prenatal diagnosis of a fetal anomaly (Lancaster 1987). Major malformations were reported in 37 fetuses and infants, resulting in an incidence of 2.2%. Six infants had spina bifida, compared with an expected number of 1.2 ($P = 0.0015$), and four infants had transposition of the great vessels compared with an expected number of 0.6 ($P = 0.0034$).

A larger series was reported by the same group in 1991. Included in the register were 5016 births and induced abortions with a malformation rate of 2.2%. Significant increases in the number of cases of spina bifida (9 observed, 3.4 expected), oesophageal atresia (6 observed, 1.4 expected), exomphalos (4 observed, 1.2 expected) and prune belly syndrome (3 observed, 0.2 expected) were found. Considering these numbers, one has to have in mind that induced abortions are included. Among infants conceived between 1979 and 1993 in Australia and New Zealand, Lancaster et al. reported a malformation rate of 2.5% for 6388 births after IVF (singletons 2.9%, multiples 1.8%) and 2.7% for 3409 births after GIFT (singletons 2.9%, multiples 2.3%) (Lancaster 1996).

In a retrospective study Beral et al. found a rate of major congenital anomalies in the first week of life of 2.2% in 1581 IVF infants (2.1% in singletons, 2.3% in twins and 2.4% in triplets) (Beral et al. 1990). A definition of major malformations was not given in this study. The malformation rate was only weakly related to multiplicity, and it was far from being significantly different between these groups.

Westergaard et al. analysed data from the Danish In Vitro Fertilisation Registry for the period 1994–1995 (Westergaard et al. 1999). A control group was generated through data from the Danish Medical Birth Registry. The control group was matched for maternal age, child's year of birth, parity and multiple pregnancies. After ART there were 1756 deliveries of 2245 children, with 24.3%

twins and 1.8% triplets. Of these, 1.3% were stillborn. Of all ART pregnancies and of pregnancies that resulted in a delivery, 13.2% and 15.4%, respectively, had an invasive prenatal diagnosis with karyotyping. Of all examined fetuses, 3.5% had an abnormal karyotype. Of all live births and stillbirths in the ART group and control group, 107 and 103 children (4.8% and 4.6%), respectively, were born with major or minor malformations (no significant difference). No definition was given for major or minor malformations in this study. The malformation rate in the background population consisting of all pregnancies and childbirths in Denmark in 1995 was stated to be 2.8%. Of the children born with malformations after ART and in the control group, 45.8% and 60.2%, respectively, belonged to multiple pregnancies. Of the 107 children with malformations, 94 were born after IVF (94/1913, 4.9%), 3 after ICSI (3/180, 1.7%), 3 after frozen embryo replacement (3/105, 2.9%) and 7 (7/47, 14.9%) after oocyte donation.

Ericson and Kallen (2001) investigated congenital malformations in infants born in Sweden after IVF during the period 1982–1997 using the Medical Birth Registry (MBR) of Sweden. They compared their data with a population-based control group (n = 1,690,577). Among all infants born after IVF, 18% were born after ICSI and 42% were born from multiple pregnancies. The presence of a congenital malformation was represented in this registry with the relevant ICD code. The survey included 9175 children born after IVF, of whom 516 were identified as having a congenital malformation (5.6%) according to the ICD code. The odds ratio (OR) when compared with the general population was 1.4 (CI 1.3–1.5). However, the excess of risk disappeared when confounders, including year of birth, maternal age, parity and period of unwanted childlessness, were taken into consideration (OR 0.89). In these calculations many mild and variable conditions were included as well as others, such as patent ductus and undescended testicles which are specifically related to preterm birth or are not considered as a malformation per se. Exclusion of these conditions and of the common and variable condition of preauricular appendix did not change the OR substantially. The OR was only 1.09 when the analysis was restricted to multiple pregnancies. For some conditions an increase in risk of about threefold was seen. These conditions included neural tube defects, alimentary atresias, omphaloceles, and, in the case of ICSI, hypospadias. No excess risk of hypospadias was seen after IVF. On the other hand no child was born with a neural tube defect after ICSI.

Some smaller series of children born after assisted reproductive techniques (ART) have also been reported. One is the study of 961 children by Rizk et al. giving a malformation rate of 2.7% among multiple pregnancies and 2.4% among singletons (Rizk et al. 1991a). Cohen et al. found 2.5% (23/938) congenital malformations among singleton births as compared with 36% (8/22) among multiple births (Cohen et al. 1988). Sunde et al. reported five major malformations (1.1%) in 433 infants born after IVF, without giving a definition of a malformation (Sunde et al. 1990). Schattman et al. reported a major malformation rate after IVF within the first year of life of 3.6% (11 of 303 children). The data were acquired by a questionnaire with a 68% response. This malformation rate is comparable to that found in the New York population (Schattman et al. 1995).

Table 7.1. Incidence of major malformations in children born after IVF

Study	Design	Total number of children	Number of children with malformations (%)
Cohen et al. 1988	Retrospective	960	31 (3.2)
Sunde et al. 1990	Retrospective	433	5 (1.1)
Beral et al. 1990	Retrospective	1581	35 (2.2)
Bonduelle et al. 1994	Prospective	55	2 (3.6)
Schattman et al. 1995	Retrospective	303	11 (3.6)
Lancaster 1996	Retrospective	9807	247 (2.5)
Lancaster 1996	Retrospective	5957	158 (2.7)
Govaerts et al. 1998	Retrospective	145	3 (2.2)
Van Golde et al. 1999	Retrospective	132	4 (3.0)
Deutsches IVF Register 2000	Retrospective	2149	26 (1.2)
Westergaard et al. 1999	Retrospective	1913	94 (4.9)
Aytoz et al. 1999	Retrospective	224	10 (5.4)
Ericson and Kallen 2001	Retrospective	9175	516 (5.6)
Hanson et al. 1985	Prospective	2995	112 (3.8)

In a prospective study by Morin et al., a cohort of 83 IVF children were compared with a group of 93 matched controls for congenital malformations (Morin et al. 1989). A general paediatric examination looked for > 130 major and minor malformations. Historical survey, physical examination, neurological examination and electrocardiography, as well as abdominal and cranial ultrasound, were performed. No association between IVF and an increased risk of congenital malformations was documented in this study. Kanyo and Konc followed 134 children born after non-contact laser-assisted hatching. They reported a malformation rate of 2.2% (Kanyo and Konc 2000).

Only recently an increase in the malformation rate of children born after conventional IVF as well as after ICSI has been reported. In a retrospective, register-based cohort study in Western Australia the authors found a twofold increased risk of both ART techniques as compared to naturally conceived children (Hansen et al. 2002). For conventional IVF, 837 children were compared to a control cohort of 4000 spontaneously conceived children. The OR for major malformation was 2.0 (95% CI 1.5–2.9) and this did not change even if several confounding factors were taken into account (Hansen et al. 2002).

A summary of the data from these studies of the incidence of major malformations in children born after IVF is presented in Table 7.1.

Congenital Malformations After ICSI

The question of a potentially increased risk of malformation again arose with the introduction of ICSI to the field of ART. Concern was expressed as to whether the selection of single sperms by a technician or a biologist would circumvent some of the biological rules of sperm selection. Furthermore, it was suggested that the ICSI technique itself might introduce an increased risk of malformation in the children, since it might lead to damage to the oocyte. On the other hand, however, patients undergoing ICSI are a special subgroup suffering from an increased risk of chromosomal abnormalities and other genetic aberrations, and may further carry an increased undefined genetic risk. Therefore, the question of malformed infants following ICSI is quite interesting, and is important in the counselling of prospective parents.

Regarding the selection of sperms, Engel et al. (1996) have clearly shown that, from a theoretical point of view, the selection of sperms by a human instead of nature does not overcome a natural selection mechanism – since such a mechanism does not exist at all. Otherwise – if the female genital tract or the oocyte itself could select against genetic abnormalities – we would not expect, for example, the transmission of autosomal recessive disorders with a calculable incidence of 25% in parents heterozygous for these alleles.

D'Hooghe et al. followed up 115 pregnancies obtained by ICSI. Two of 98 ongoing pregnancies were terminated after prenatal diagnosis of a malformation. The major malformation rate of 115 infants was 4.3% (5/115) (D'Hooghe et al. 2000). Antoni and Hamori analysed neonatal and paediatric data from the paediatric follow-up of 1290 children conceived by ICSI. They found a major malformation rate of 3.4% (44/1290). Major malformations affected the cardiovascular system more frequently then any other organ system. They also found that boys showed a 2.5-fold higher incidence of major malformations than girls (14/650, 2.1%, in girls; 30/640, 4.7%, in boys; $P < 0.025$) (Antoni and Hamori 2001).

In a retrospective study, Bajirova et al. compared the malformation rate in pregnancies achieved by ICSI using epididymal spermatozoa ($n = 546$) and those using testicular spermatozoa ($n = 201$). Data were obtained from the French IVF register (FIVNAT). The malformation rate in full-term infants and therapeutic abortions was 6.5% with testicular spermatozoa and 2.4% with epididymal spermatozoa, a significant difference (Bajirova et al. 2001).

Westergard et al. reported a malformation rate of 1.7% (3/149) after ICSI but this was not significantly lower than after other techniques of ART in their survey. However, this represents only a small sample size as Danish clinics began their ICSI programmes around 1995 (Westergaard et al. 1999). Sutcliffe et al. compared 221 naturally conceived children with 208 children conceived after ICSI in a prospective, controlled and standardized study. The number of children with major congenital malformation was comparable after ICSI (4.8%) and spontaneous conception (4.5%) (Sutcliffe et al. 2001). The German IVF Register (Deutsches IVF Register 2000) recorded a malformation rate of 2.05% (42/2599).

Another example of a large registry on malformations following ART is the ESHRE task force on ICSI. It collects data from centres worldwide. Again, no standardization of follow-up or malformation classification is done, and no data are available on the completeness of malformation registration. Again, however, this registry provides follow-up data over a number of years and therefore helps to detect possible trends. Furthermore, the large number of cases helps to answer questions regarding the effectiveness and safety of ICSI.

For the years 1993–1994, the ESHRE task force on ICSI (Tarlatzis 1996) has reported the incidence of congenital malformations, In 763 infants born after the use of ejaculated spermatozoa there were 17 major (2.2%) and 108 minor (14.1%) malformations, in 36 infants born after the use of epididymal spermatozoa there were one major (2.8%) and two minor (5.5%) malformations, and in 8 infants born after the use of testicular spermatozoa there were no malformations. In the year 1995 the ESHRE task force on ICSI (Tarlatzis and Bili 1998) in 2486 infants born after the use of ejaculated spermatozoa noted 47 (1.9%) major and 185 minor (7.4%) malformations, in 119 children born after the use of epididymal spermatozoa noted no major and 3 (2.5%) minor malformations and in 63 children born after the use of testicular spermatozoa noted 3 major (4.8%) and 2 minor (3.2%) malformations. The ESHRE task force considered major malformations as those causing functional impairment or requiring surgical correction; all others were classified as minor.

Wennerholm et al. studied the rate of congenital malformations in a cohort of children born after ICSI using the Swedish Medical Birth Registry (MBR) and the Registry of Congenital Malformations (RCM). All stillborn and live-born infants delivered after 28 weeks of gestation were included. Induced abortions were excluded. Malformations were defined according to the International Classification of Diseases (ICD-9, ICD-10). In the study, 1139 infants born in Sweden after 937 ICSI procedures in two IVF clinics in Gothenburg from 1993 to 1998 were examined. The total number of infants with an identified anomaly was 87 (7.6%), of whom 40 were showed a mild or variable condition (Wennerholm et al. 2000b). The authors found that a substantial number of congenital malformations were not included in the MBR. This illustrates the problems in evaluating data obtained by screening of medical records for selected patients, e.g. infants born after IVF or ICSI. Rates of malformations obtained in this manner are difficult to compare with rates determined from population registers. However, even after restricting the conditions identified to those reported in the MBR, an increased risk was seen in children born after ICSI. For ICSI children, the OR for having any major or minor malformation was 1.75 (95% CI 1.19–2.58) after stratification for delivery hospital, year of birth and maternal age. Relatively serious malformations were more common in twins than in singletons. If stratification for singletons and twins was also done, the OR was reduced to 1.19 (95% CI 0.79–1.81) and no difference was obvious any longer.

To a large extent, the excess risk can be explained by conditions associated with multiple and premature birth, notable patent ductus arteriosus and undescended testicles. It is also plausible that paediatric examination and recording of data concerning infants born after IVF and ICSI may have been more detailed compared to that for infants born after spontaneous conception. The only specific malformation that was found to occur in excess in children born after ICSI, even after control for multiples, was hypospadias (relative risk 3.0, 95% CI 1.09–6.50). When specific malformations were compared between infants born after IVF and after ICSI, there were no neural tube defects or hydrocephaly observed among children born after ICSI but an over-representation among those born after IVF, even though this difference may have been random.

These conditions are associated with twinning, and the rate of twin pregnancies after IVF was higher (27%) than after ICSI (20%) (Wennerholm et al. 2000b).

The group of Van Steirteghem and coworkers, mainly Dr. Bonduelle from Brussels, have performed a prospective study on children born after ICSI. A standardized and prospective design was used, since all examination procedures were defined in a study protocol before. Data collection included physical examination at birth, and at 2 and 12 months of age and was done by a neonatologist who was also trained in medical genetics. However, major malformations were not classified according to an internationally accepted malformation catalogue, but defined as causing functional impairment or requiring surgical correction. This has been criticized by others in the recent literature (Kurinczuk and Bower 1997). The Brussels series of children born after ICSI is meanwhile, however, the largest and surely the most important published series. First, this group (Bonduelle et al. 1994) published data of 55 children, 21 born after replacement of SUZI embryos and 24 after replacement of ICSI embryos, 10 after replacement of a combination of SUZI and ICSI embryos; two major (3.6%) and six minor (10.9%) malformations were noted.

The largest cohort published so far in a journal, is that of 2889 children (Bonduelle et al. 2002), 2955 live-born and 40 stillborn children, 1499 singletons and 1341 multiples after ICSI. Of these children, 2477 were born after ICSI with ejaculated sperm, 105 after ICSI with epididymal sperm, 206 with testicular sperm, and 52 with donated sperm. A total of 96 major malformations (3.38%) defined as those causing functional impairment or requiring surgical correction were observed among the live births. Of 1499 singleton children and 1341 multiples, 46 (3.06%) and 50 (3.65%), respectively, had a major malformation. If affected live births, stillbirths and induced abortions for malformations are all included, the malformation rate was 4.22%. Compared to a similarly evaluated cohort of children born after conventional IVF, the malformation rate was not increased (4.66%).

The malformation rates in different subgroups of this survey were 3.3% (3/90) in cases of ICSI with epididymal spermatozoa, 1.6% (2/118) in the testicular spermatozoa group and 1.3% (1/78) in the children born after replacement of frozen/thawed supernumerary embryos after ICSI (Bonduelle et al. 1998c). As the totals in these subgroups are still low, it is difficult to reach a conclusion concerning any differences due to the origin of the sperm, but there appears to be no particular reason for concern.

A special case might be the use of immature spermatozoa. Spermatid microinjection into oocytes has been applied in cases of ICSI in which no spermatozoa could be found in numerous testicular samples. Al-Hasani et al. were the first worldwide to report on two pregnancies resulting from elongated spermatid injection form frozen-thawed testicular tissue (Al Hasani et al. 1999). Until now, just a small number of infants have been born after injection of round (ROSI) or elongated (ELSI) spermatids. There is much doubt as to whether ROSI has any benefit at all in ICSI cycles: experiments in non-human primate models have shown no fertilization (Hewitson et al. 2000). Others have shown fertilization in the human with the use of ROSI, but a blastocyst formation of only

7.6%. After transfer of blastocysts in 12 patients no pregnancies could be achieved (Urman et al. 2002).

Zech et al. have reported two cases of malformations out of four pregnancies obtained after ELSI retrieved from patients suffering from non-obstructive azoospermia (Zech et al. 2000). The first case consisted of a hydrocephalus diagnosed by ultrasound in week 20 of gestation. The fetal karyotype showed a trisomy 9. The other malformation observed was an open lumbosacral myelomeningocele, interpreted as Arnold Chiari syndrome type II with a normal male karyotype. However, these numbers have to be interpreted more as case reports than as a representative cohort of children.

Since the number of children born after ROSI and ELSI is still quite small, and no further series have been reported, no conclusions can be drawn, since both anomalies have also been observed after spontaneous conception and in IVF with or without ICSI. It is not yet known if spermatid injection itself or the basic cause of infertility in these male patients or an unknown genetic disposition might have caused these anomalies (Al Hasani et al. 1999).

However, the definition of major and minor malformations is of critical importance. This becomes clear with a good example from literature data. Thus, by the definition used by Bonduelle et al. and by the EHRE task force, major malformations are those that generally cause functional impairment or require surgical correction (Bonduelle et al. 1995a,b, 1996b, 1998a). Kurinczuk and Bower using the British Paediatric Association's ICD-9 system recalculated the incidence of major malformations reported by Bonduelle et al. and found it to be significantly increased (Bonduelle et al. 1996b; Kurinczuk and Bower 1997). Kurinczuk and Bower reanalysed data of 420 live-born infants conceived by ICSI in Belgium and 100,454 live born infants in Western Australia delivered during the same period. Bonduelle et al. had given a rate of major congenital malformations for this cohort of 3.3%. Reanalysing these data Kurinczuk and Bower found a major malformation rate of 7.28% and a rate of 0.71% for minor malformations. Therefore, they state that infants born after ICSI were twice as likely as Western Australian infants to have a major birth defect (OR 2.03, 95% CI 1.40–2.93, $P = 0.0002$) and nearly 50% more likely to have a minor birth defect (OR 1.49, 95% CI 0.48–4.66, $P = 0.49$). However, although the same classification system is applied to both cohorts, differences in malformation rates may be a result of differences in the way the data were obtained. The Belgium group conducted a prospective study in which the data were obtained in a standardized fashion by a trained paediatrician, while the Australian National Perinatal Statistics data were obtained in a non-standardized passive fashion. Malformation rates are likely to be underestimated in registers where reliance is placed on routine notifications that are not backed up by verifications from other sources.

However, as pointed out here, as well as by Bonduelle et al. in their response to the reanalysis of the Australian data, the higher rate was probably due to the different definition as well as the overestimation of certain transient cardiac defects in ICSI infants due to extensive investigations (Bonduelle et al. 1998a).

Finally, recent data do point to a higher malformation rate in register-based studies. With all the drawbacks of those studies – e.g. a reporting bias regarding malformations – these data have to be taken into account when the malformation rate in these children is discussed. In two Swedish studies the risk of hypospadias was significantly increased in children born after ICSI with an OR of 3.0 (95 % CI 1.09–6.50) (Wennerholm et al. 2000a) and 1.35 (95 % CI 1.19–1.56) (Ericson and Kallen 2001).

Others have described an overall increased risk. In the study discussed above by Hansen et al. from Western Australia, a comparison of 301 children born after ICSI and 4000 spontaneously conceived children showed an increased malformation risk after ICSI (OR 2.0, 95 % CI 1.3–3.2) (Hansen et al. 2002). This was the same as the result for conventional IVF. Even if these were the first results showing a real increased risk of malformations after ICSI, the data have to be confirmed in further, preferably prospective, controlled studies.

Risk figures in national and international registries, such as the German IVF Registry or the ESHRE Task Force on ICSI, will probably be somewhat lower, as it is unlikely that malformations are generally looked for and reported as carefully as in a prospective survey. Data obtained through standard data collection forms are mostly filled in at birth. The children born after assisted reproduction and those born after spontaneous conception are not examined in a systematic manner and follow-up data are usually not acquired. There is no system to check the results reported or for missing data.

Table 7.2. Incidence of major malformations in children born after ICSI

Study	Design	Total number of children	Number of children with malformations (%)
Bonduelle et al. 1998c	Prospective	848	23 (2.7)
Bonduelle et al. 1995a	Prospective	273	6 (2.2)
Govaerts et al. 1995	Retrospective	76	3 (3.9)
Tarlatzis 1996	Prospective	807	18 (2.2)
Chandley et al. 1975	Retrospective	210	2 (1.0)
Bonduelle et al. 1996b	Prospective	877	23 (2.6)
Govaerts et al. 1998	Retrospective	145	4 (2.8)
Tarlatzis and Bili 1998	Prospective	2668	50 (1.9)
Bonduelle et al. 1998a	Prospective	1966	46 (2.3)
Palermo et al. 1996	Retrospective	1131	23 (2.0)
Loft et al. 1999	Retrospective	730	16 (2.2)
Ludwig et al. 1999c	Prospective	267	9 (3.4)
Deutsches IVF Register 2000	Retrospective	2599	42 (2.1)
Sutcliffe et al. 1999	Retrospective	123	6 (4.9)
Van Golde et al. 1999	Retrospective	120	2 (1.7)
Aytoz et al. 1999	Retrospective	166	4 (2.4)
Wennerholm et al. 2000b	Retrospective	1139	87 (7.6)
Ericson and Kallen 2001[a]	Retrospective	9175	516 (5.6)
Nielsen and Wohlert 1991	Retrospective	1290	44 (3.4)
Hanson et al. 1985	Prospective	2899	96 (3.4)

[a] Ericson and Kallen (2001) included children born after IVF and after ICSI.

Table 7.3. Results form the EHRE task force (Tarlatzis 1996; Tarlatzis and Bili 1998) for 1993–1994 and 1995 and from Bonduelle et al. (1998c) regarding the malformation rate depending on the sperm's origin

Study	Origin of sperm	Total number of children	Number of children with malformations (%)
Tarlatzis 1996	Ejaculated	763	17 (2.2)
	Epididymal	36	1 (2.7)
	Testicular	8	0
Tarlatzis and Bili 1998	Ejaculated	2486	47 (1.9)
	Epididymal	119	0
	Testicular	63	3 (4.8)
Bonduelle et al. 1998c	Ejaculated	1699	40 (2.3)
	Epididymal	90	3 (3.3)
	Testicular	118	2 (1.6)
Ogura and Yanagimachi 1995	Epididymal	546	(2.4)
	Testicular	201	(6.5)

A summary of the data from studies of the incidence of major malformations in children born after ICSI is presented in Table 7.2, and a summary of the results of studies regarding the malformation rate depending on the sperm's origin is presented in Table 7.3.

Congenital Malformations After SUZI

In a retrospective study Patrat et al. investigated 50 pregnancies obtained by SUZI during the period 1991–1994. Of those pregnancies, 7 (14%) ended in a clinical abortion and 2 (4%) were ectopic. Among the 41 resulting ongoing pregnancies, the discovery of one anencephaly led to a medical abortion. Thus, 40 deliveries including 6 twin pregnancies occurred, leading to the births of 45 live neonates and 1 stillbirth. Two children (4.3%) showed a malformation: the first one had one thumb with congenital shelf and the second a polymalformative neurological syndrome (Patrat et al. 1999).

Bonduelle et al. followed 163 couples who underwent SUZI or ICSI in a prospective study that included a prenatal diagnosis and clinical follow-up of the children. In 23 pregnancies occurring after SUZI, 15 women gave birth to 21 children. After replacement of combined SUZI and ICSI embryos, ten pregnancies resulted in eight deliveries of ten infants. Transfer of ICSI embryos led to 130 pregnancies ending in 20 deliveries of 24 infants, with many others still ongoing at that time. In total, 55 children were examined: 29 boys and 26 girls. One child from a singleton pregnancy showed multiple congenital malformations; one twin child showed a quadriparesis. In this observational study on a limited number of children, the incidence of major malformations was not different from the incidence in the general population (Bonduelle et al. 1994).

Congenital Malformations After GIFT or Intrauterine Insemination

Meirow and Schenker evaluated data relating to GIFT from world reports, national registers and a meta-analysis of medical publications during the years 1986–1991. Among 10,667 clinical pregnancies reported, the malformation rate was calculated to be 2.8% (Meirow and Schenker 1995). Among infants conceived between 1979 and 1993 in Australia and New Zealand, Lancaster (1996) give a malformation rate of 2.7% for 3409 GIFT births (singletons 2.9%, multiples 2.3%).

Regarding the malformation rate after intrauterine insemination, only limited numbers are available. Sunde et al. reported one major malformation in 127 (0.8%) pregnancies achieved by intrauterine insemination (Sunde et al. 1990).

Amuzu et al. evaluated the pregnancies of 427 women who conceived through artificial insemination by donor (AID) over a 12-year period. Follow-up was completed on 481 children, among whom 22 major (4.6%) and 38 minor (7.9%) malformations were found. No definition of major and minor malformations was given (Amuzu et al. 1990). Grefestette et al. described the outcome of 487 pregnancies achieved by AID. The malformation rate in this cohort was 3.4%. A definition of malformation was not given (Grefenstette et al. 1990). Lansac et al. followed 620 pregnancies after AID with a non-defined malformation rate of 1.5% (Lansac et al. 1997).

Thepot et al. evaluated 11,535 pregnancies obtained by AID, which resulted in 9794 live births and 41 medically induced abortions. Malformations were classified according to the World Health Organization international classification system (ICD-9). The total frequency of birth defects was 1.7% ($n = 165$). Single malformations accounted for 1.2% ($n = 118$). In order of decreasing frequency, the malformations found affected the cardiovascular system, the limbs and the urinary system (Thepot et al. 1996).

Congenital Malformations After Cryopreservation

Cryopreservation and thawing involve major cellular changes and it is not clear whether they have adverse effects for the offspring. There is no evidence that freezing itself is mutagenic. However, it has been suggested that the cumulative effect of background radiation may increase the mutation rate, since no DNA repair will occur at the temperature of liquid nitrogen (Biggers 1981).

Frydman et al. have described the obstetric outcome of 28 pregnancies (including 3 twin pregnancies) resulting from cryopreserved embryos (Frydman et al. 1989). There was no matched control group. Apart from one major limb malformation all children were born healthy. Therefore, the malformation rate could be calculated as 3.2%.

In a retrospective study, Wada et al. found that the prevalence of congenital malformations was smaller in the cryopreserved group (1%) than the group using fresh embryos (3%, $p < 0.05$) (Wada et al. 1994). Sutcliffe et al. retrospectively studied the perinatal outcome among 91 children from cryopreserved

embryos directly after birth (Sutcliffe et al. 1995a,b). Compared with 83 spontaneously conceived children, the malformation rate was 31.9% versus 21.7% for
minor malformations and 3.3% versus 2.4% for major malformations, respectively. There were no statistically significant differences.

In an observational follow-up study, Heijnsbroek et al. evaluated the pregnancy outcome of the first 30 women who conceived after transfer of cryopreserved embryos. No major malformation was found (Heijnsbroek et al. 1995).
Olivennes et al. analysed the perinatal outcome of 82 children born after cryopreservation and found a congenital malformation rate of 3.4%; no control group
was employed (Olivennes et al. 1996).

Wennerholm et al. compared 270 children born from cryopreserved embryos
with an equal number of children born after the transfer of fresh embryos
(Wennerholm et al. 1997). The malformation rate in children born after the
transfer of cryopreserved embryos was 2.7% (7/270) which was not different
from the rate following the transfer of fresh embryos. In 1998 Bonduelle et al.
reported a follow-up study of 48 pregnancies after replacement of previously
cryopreserved ICSI embryos (Bonduelle et al. 1998c). They observed one child
born with a major malformation in this cohort. In the follow-up examinations at
2 months and at 1 year, no additional anomalies were observed.

In frozen IVF cycles, Aytoz et al. found a major malformation in 4 of 165
infants (2.4%) and in the fresh embryo cycles in 10 of 224 infants (4.5%) (Aytoz
et al. 1999). In frozen ICSI cycles they observed a major malformation in 3 of
104 infants (2.9%), while they found a malformation in 4 of 166 infants (2.4%)
in the fresh ICSI group. Major malformations were defined according to the
definition used by Bonduelle et al. and the ESHRE task force.

In the German IVF Registry the reported malformation rate was 1.37%
(6/438) in children born after using cryopreserved embryos (DIR 1999), and
is again in the same range as that for children born using cells not previously
cryopreserved (Deutsches IVF Register 2000). The ESHRE task force on ICSI

Table 7.4. Incidence of major malformations in children born after the transfer of cryopreserved embryos

Study	Design	Total number of children	Number of children with malformations (%)
Frydman et al. 1989	Retrospective	31	1 (3.2)
Wada et al. 1994	Retrospective	283	3 (1.0)
Sutcliffe et al. 1995b	Retrospective	91	3 (3.3)
Heijnsbroek et al. 1995	Retrospective	30	0
Olivennes et al. 1996	Retrospective	82	3 (3.4)
Wennerholm et al. 1997	Retrospective	270	7 (2.2)
Bonduelle et al. 1998c	Prospective	48	1 (2.1)
Tarlatzis and Bili 1998	Retrospective	139	3 (2.2)
Deutsches IVF Register 2000	Retrospective	438	6 (1.4)
Aytoz et al. 1999	Retrospective	169	7 (4.1)

reported 3 major (2.2%) and 2 minor (9.3%) malformations in 139 children born after using frozen-thawed ICSI embryos (Tarlatzis and Bili 1998).

The number of studies on the effect of cryopreservation on human embryos is limited, and the number of children studied is rather small. So far, however, there is no evidence from human data on cryopreservation indicating a risk for the offspring (Table 7.4).

An Increased Risk for Certain Malformations

Some malformations have been reported by several investigators to be increased after ART treatment. These are discussed in the following section. However, one has to take into account that in comparison to the controls the overall risk in all these studies was always similar, and that the elevated risk was either caused by overestimation due to a more intensive follow-up of these children, or by over-reporting. Therefore, especially due to the point that the finding of these anomalies was not consistently described in all the studies, a specific malformation prevalence seems not to be present. Case reports are not included as they are shown separately (Table 7.5).

Neural Tube Defects

An association between neural tube defects and ovarian stimulation has been described and the possibility of an increased risk after IVF has also been mentioned (Lancaster et al. 2000). The relative risk reported by Ericson and Kallen (2001) is 2.9 for neural tube defects (95% CI 1.5–5.1). Of 12 infants with neural tube defects identified after IVF, 9 were born from multiple pregnancies. Among 1694 live births and stillbirths and 3 terminations of pregnancy after IVF, Lancaster et al. observed 6 infants with spina bifida compared with an expected number of 1.2 ($P = 0.0015$) (Lancaster 1987). While the overall incidence of

Table 7.5. Case reports regarding malformations in children born after ART

Report	Syndrome	Method
Yovich et al. 1987	Goldenhar	ICSI
Hsiung et al. 1987	Down	IVF
Marino and Marcelletti 1989	Pulmonary atresia	IVF
Tejada et al. 1990	Monosomy 4q31	GIFT
Cummins and Jequier 1994	Baller-Gerold	IVF
Shozu et al. 1997	Meckel-Grüber	IVF
Whitman-Elia et al. 1997	Oesophageal atresia	IVF
Strain et al. 1998	True hermaphrodite chimera	IVF
Ferraris et al. 1999	Goldenhar	IVF
Zech et al. 2000	Trisomy 9, hydrocephalus	ICSI/ELSI
	Arnold Chiari type II	ICSI/ELSI

major malformations (2.2%) after IVF in this study was similar to that in the general population, the incidence of spina bifida was significantly increased. Three of these six infants with spina bifida were born from multiple pregnancies. In 1991 Lancaster reported data on 5016 births and induced abortions. In this cohort, the incidence of spina bifida was also increased (9 cases observed, 3.4 cases expected) (Lancaster 1987). On the other hand Ericson and Kallen (2001) did not observe a single case of spina bifida in their detailed analysis of 9175 children born after IVF and ICSI. Wennerhom et al. also found no children born with spina bifida after ICSI in their sample (Wennerholm et al. 2000b). As most pregnant women have prenatal ultrasound, anencephaly is nearly always detected. Those born are usually members of a twin pair, one infant with an anencephaly and the other normal. Twin pregnancies with an anencephalic twin are often interrupted.

Alimentary Tract Atresia

Another group of malformations which has been found to occur at an increased rate after IVF in some studies is alimentary tract atresia: oesophageal, small bowel and anal atresia. Such an association has been reported by Lancaster (1989). Ericson and Kallen (2001) observed a two- to threefold increased rate (Ericson and Kallen 2001). The risk of alimentary tract atresia in twins seems to have been increased about three times but this was mainly associated with monozygotic twinning (Harris et al. 1995). In a cohort of 5016 births and induced abortions, Lancaster observed 6 cases of oesophageal atresia compared to an expected number of 1.4. Therefore, there is not a great difference between the observed number and the expected number of infants born after IVF and with an atresia (Kallen et al. 1991).

Hypospadias

Hypospadias or incomplete development of the anterior urethra is a common genitourinary birth defect that occurs in approximately 0.3% of live births (Barros et al. 1997). The increased incidence of hypospadias after IVF may indicate that fetal endocrine abnormalities are more common in couples with a history of infertility. Alternatively, it may indicate that drugs given as part of the IVF protocol may disturb the maternal-fetal endocrine milieu. An increased risk of hypospadias after IVF has previously been reported. It has been reported to be associated with progesterone treatment (Barros et al. 1997).

As a consequence of progestin administration fetal dihydrotestosterone levels may be reduced during a critical period of urethral development (weeks 8–13). Although this theory appears reasonable, a prospective study by Mau et al. showed that progestin intake during pregnancy does not contribute significantly to the risk of hypospadias (Mau 1981). Other possible aetiologies include maternal endocrine abnormalities that may be present more commonly in infertile couples. There are also others who do not believe that progesterone treatment causes hypospadias (Kallen et al. 1991, 1992).

To assess the risk of hypospadias after IVF, Silver et al. analysed data from 1988 to 1992 retrospectively (Silver et al. 1999). Their data indicated a fivefold increase of hypospadias after IVF, with an incidence of 1.5% in the IVF group and 0.3% in the control group ($P < 0.001$). A tendency was noted in the IVF group for a family history of hypospadias and infertility, not including the couple who underwent IVF, but this tendency did not reach statistical significance. Macnab and Zouves reported an incidence of 3.8% in boys conceived by IVF compared to 0.27% in their control group (Macnab and Zouves 1991). The data presented by Ericson and Kallen who observed only an increased risk with ICSI (relative risk 1.5, 95% CI 1.0–2.1) suggest that the increased risk for hypospadias is specific for ICSI (Ericson and Kallen 2001). This was confirmed by Wennerholm et al., who reported a relative risk of 3.0 for infants born after ICSI (95% CI 1.09–6.50) (Wennerholm et al. 2000b).

Hypospadias have been shown to be associated with paternal subfertility (Kallen et al. 1991), and this would explain the specific association with ICSI. An increased occurrence of testicular anomalies has been described in fathers of hypospadic boys (Sweet et al. 1974). A possible explanation is the transfer of a gene from father to son which causes testicular impairment as early as fetal stages, resulting in an increased risk of hypospadias. In the father the same gene may cause subfertility.

Conclusion

Theoretically, birth defects after IVF may be increased because of the induction of chromosomal aberrations, an increase in fertilization rate by abnormal spermatozoa or the influence of possible physical or chemical teratogens. However, most studies up to now do not support these theories.

A number of authors have studied the occurrence of birth defects in children born after IVF. The number of newborns studied ranged from fewer than 100 to several thousand. Most of these studies found an increased risk of malformations compared with the general population. Some studies showed an increased prevalence of certain malformations such as spina bifida, alimentary tract atresia or hypospadias in children born after IVF. These findings have not been confirmed by others and may be explained by some weakness in the studies:

- Most of the data were derived from retrospective studies.
- These studies often use a different study design for children born after ART and for those born after spontaneous conception.
- Some studies did not include a control group. In those studies including a control group, children born after assisted reproduction and those born after spontaneous conception were often not examined in a systematic manner, especially if the control group was taken from national birth registers.

- Comparing different studies, the underlying definition of a malformation has to be taken into account. Some studies include therapeutic abortions while other studies only include live born and stillborn infants with a certain (and varying) birth weight.

These variations in study design explain the difficulties when comparing data from different studies and the impossibility of giving an exact malformation rate associated with a certain technique or even with spontaneous conception.

In a very recent register-based study, a twofold increased malformation risk for children born after ICSI as well as after conventional IVF has been found (Hansen et al. 2002). Despite an excellent design, this analysis was retrospective and strategies to exclude the possibility of an over-reporting bias in the ART groups may not have been sufficient. However, these numbers are important and have to be taken into account for future counselling of IVF and ICSI patients.

As with other risks, associated with early abortion, ectopic and heterotopic pregnancies and pregnancy course, potential parents have to be counselled about the risks they carry individually, e.g. a higher age or certain genetic factors – and about a genetic background risk associated with infertility.

8 Perinatal Outcome and Follow-up of Children Born from ART

Georgine Huber, Michael Ludwig

The widespread application of new reproduction techniques has led to concern not only about the course of such pregnancies but also about the offspring's health and postnatal development.

Several studies have been reported examining the incidence of chromosomal anomalies, congenital malformations and child development after assisted reproduction. Lancaster states that advanced parental age (chromosomal abnormalities with advanced maternal age and point mutations with advanced paternal age), underlying causes of infertility, drugs such as clomiphene and IVF procedures (e.g. freezing and thawing) are factors that might influence the risk of chromosomal abnormalities and congenital malformations (Lancaster 1985). The high incidence of multiple births with the risk of prematurity and adverse health outcomes such as low birth weight, respiratory distress syndrome, need for ventilation, intraventricular haemorrhage or retinopathy, might seriously endanger the offspring's postnatal development. The literature on the health and development of these children is reviewed in this chapter. For a better understanding of the data, we have subdivided the presentation into non-controlled and controlled studies.

Descriptive Studies Without Control Groups

Yovich et al. assessed the development of the first 20 infants resulting from IVF in Western Australia at their first birthday, including one pair of twins and two sets of triplets (Yovich et al. 1986). Their development status was measured on the Griffith Development Scales for children. All infants had progressed normally, and for five test scales their developmental assessment was in advance of the mean rates. The authors point out, however, that it cannot be concluded that these children had advanced development, as a control series was not studied.

A non-controlled study by Mushin et al. examined 33 children resulting from IVF aged between 12 and 37 months as to their early psychosocial development which was assessed using the Bayley Scales of Infant Development (Mushin et al. 1986). Overall scores were within the normal range and problems presented were in accordance with the high incidence of prematurity (21.2%) and twins (36.4%) in the studied group of children.

Wennerholm et al. performed a follow-up of 95 children resulting from IVF-ET from 18 months up to 8 years (Wennerholm et al. 1991). Of the 95 children,

Table 8.1. Perinatal outcome and follow-up of children born after ART. Descriptive studies without control groups

Study	No. of children	ART	Age of children (months)	Tests	Results
Yovich et al. 1986	20	IVF	12	Griffith Scales	No difference
Mushin et al. 1986	33	IVF	12–37	Bayley Scales	No difference
Wennerholm et al. 1991	95	IVF	18	Physical development	Long-term sequelae associated with immaturity/birth weight

88 appeared completely healthy and normally developed, and had achieved normal height and weight within the normal Swedish range. Clear indications of disability were found in four children at follow-up. These included cerebral palsy and severe mental retardation, problems with vision, developmental delay and renal failure. In three of these children the problems were related to preterm birth and complicated neonatal history. Three more children showed borderline speech development. Long-term sequelae were associated with immaturity and low birth weight, whereas no problems were disclosed in children with an uneventful neonatal period.

A summary of these data is presented in Table 8.1.

Controlled Studies

Morin et al. found no difference in a matched study of 83 children resulting from IVF. Matching was done for age of the infant, multiple conceptions, sex, race and maternal age. The study included a control group of 93 infants, all aged between 13 and 30 months. The risks of developmental delay as assessed by the Bayley Scales were evaluated (Morin et al. 1989). Similarly, Brandes et al. studied 116 children aged between 12 and 45 months conceived by IVF and compared them with a control group matched for gestational age, multiple pregnancy and maternal characteristics, using the Bayley Scales and the Stanfort Binet Scales: development did not differ between the two groups (Brandes et al. 1992).

In a prospective follow-up study, Ron-El et al. compared the development of 30 children born after long-acting gonadotropin-releasing hormone agonist (GnRHa) treatment with that of 30 singleton infants conceived spontaneously (Ron-El et al. 1994). The General Cognitive Index demonstrated no difference between the study and the control group children who were at least 28 months old at the time of examination.

Saunders et al. used a case-matched control study in which 314 children (196 singletons, 47 sets of twins, 8 sets of triplets) conceived by IVF and 150 control infants (13 singletons, 17 sets of twins, 1 set of triplets) conceived spontaneously were compared at the age of 2 years (Saunders et al. 1996). Matching was done for multiple birth, gestation and date of birth. There was no significant inter-action between IVF status and growth or physical outcome of children when matched for plurality and gestation. Poor outcomes, for example evidence of spastic diplegia, were related to the effects of multiple births.

The development, as measured using the Griffith Scale, and behaviour, as measured using the Child Behaviour Check List, of children born after IVF was examined in a study by Cederblad et al. in which 99 children aged 33–85 months were compared with a control population (Cederblad et al. 1996). Among the study group, 34% of infants were part of a multiple birth and 28% were born prematurely. Both the IVF group as a whole and the preterm group had scores comparable with the normal population group. Children resulting from IVF who had experienced normal conditions had higher developmental quotients on the Griffith Scale than those who had been born prematurely.

Bonduelle et al. followed up 201 children from ICSI and 131 children from IVF prospectively at 2 years of age in terms of their mental development as assessed using Bayley tests (Bonduelle et al. 1998b). The results from the study groups were compared with normal values from the Dutch general population, and similar scores were shown between the study and control groups.

Van Golde et al. retrospectively analysed the physical and mental devel-opment of 132 children born after IVF and of 120 infants born after ICSI between the ages of 6 and 18 months (Van Golde et al. 1999). Follow-up data were compared with the Catalan National Developmental Scale. Measurement of weights and lengths showed no significant difference between the two groups, nor did physical or mental development.

Lahat et al. observed neurodevelopmental abnormalities in four of six children who were born after inadvertent administration of a GnRHa in early pregnancy and were compared with 20 matched controls resulting from IVF and from spontaneous pregnancies (Lahat et al. 1999). The children were examined at a mean age of 7.8 ± 2.0 years. Abnormalities included epileptic disorder, attention deficit hyperactivity disorder, motor difficulties and speech difficul-ties. Following these results the authors of this long-term follow-up emphasized that more studies are needed in children previously exposed to GnRHa before drawing any conclusions. This study, however, is the first to show abnormalities in children born after accidental administration of GnRHa in early pregnancy. Many other case reports, but with a lower quality of follow-up, as recently re-viewed, have not confirmed these observations (Cahill 1998).

Papaligoura et al. compared the mental and psychomotor development of infants conceived after ICSI treatment to infants conceived after IVF treatment (Papaligoura et al. 2001). The control group comprised infants conceived natural-ly. Each group consisted of 40 children aged between 12 and 14 months. The Bayley Scales for Infant Development were applied for assessment, and showed no significant differences between the three groups regarding mental or motor development.

A prospective longitudinal study by Place and Englert showed similar results (Place and Englert 2001). Singleton children born after ICSI ($n = 112$) were com-

Table 8.2. Perinatal outcome and follow-up of children born following ART. Controlled studies

Study	Study group		Control group	Age of children	Test	Results
	No. of children	ART	No. of children			
Morin et al. 1989	83	IVF	93 Spontaneously conceived	13–30 months	Bayley Scales	No difference
Brandes et al. 1992	116	IVF	Population control	12–45 months	Bayley Stanfort-Binet	No difference
Ron-El et al. 1994	30	GnRHa	30 Spontaneously conceived	>28 months	General Cognitive Index	No difference
Saunders et al. 1996	314	IVF	150 Spontaneously conceived	24 months	Physical development	No difference (poor outcome associated with multiples)
Cederblad et al. 1996	99	IVF	Population control	33–85 months	Griffith Scales	No difference
Bonduelle et al. 1998	201	ICSI	131 IVF	24 months	Bayley Scales	No difference
Van Golde et al. 1999	132	IVF	120 ICSI	6–18 months	Catalan National Developmental Scale	No difference
Lahat et al. 1999	6	GnRHa	20 IVF/spontaneously conceived	7.8±2.0 years	Neurodevelopmental tests	Abnormalities in four of six children
Papaligoura et al. 2001	40	ICSI	40/40 IVF/spontaneously conceived	12–14 months	Bayley Scales	No difference
Place and Englert 2001	112	ICSI	82/97 IVF/spontaneously conceived	9 months/ 18 months/ 3 years/ 5 years	Brunet-Lézine Wechsler	No difference
Sutcliff et al. 2001	208	ICSI	221 Spontaneously conceived	12–24 months	Griffith Scales	No difference

pared with a matched control group of children born after IVF (n = 82) and with children spontaneously conceived (n = 97). Matching was done for birth date, age and sex of the child, age of the mother, social class and family size. The infants were examined at the ages of 9 months, 18 months, 3 years and 5 years. The Brunet-Lézine Revised Scale was used to evaluate psychomotor development and the Wechsler Preschool and Primary Scale of Intelligence was applied to evaluate intellectual development. There were no significant differences between the three groups as to developmental or intelligence quotients.

Sutcliff et al. compared 208 singleton children born after ICSI with 221 single-ton infants conceived spontaneously in a matched case-control study of neuro-development (Sutcliffe et al. 2001). Assessment was done using the Griffith Scales. Matching included social class, maternal education level, region, sex and race. At the time of evaluation the children were between 12 and 24 months of age. No difference between the study children and their controls was found as to developmental scoring on the Griffith Scales.

A summary of these data is presented in Table 8.2.

Follow-up of Children From Cryopreserved Embryos

The number of studies following up children conceived from cryopreserved embryos is limited. So far, no evidence exists that this procedure may carry risks for the fetus or for the long-term development of the infants.

The outcome of children conceived from cryopreserved embryos was studied by Sutcliffe et al. (1995b). The development of a cohort of 91 infants from cryo-preserved embryos and 83 control children conceived spontaneously was assess-ed. The Griffith Scales of mental development were applied for evaluation. The controls were similar in age, sex and social class. At the time of examination the infants in the cryopreservation group were 25.08 months old and those in the control group were 29.19 months old. There was no evidence of developmental delay in children conceived from cryopreserved embryos compared with infants conceived spontaneously.

Olivennes et al. examined a group of 89 children aged 1–9 years conceived from cryopreserved embryos (Olivennes et al. 1996). No control group was included. To assess the development of the children < 5 years old, a questionnaire was adapted from standardized tests. The children > 5 years old were assessed in terms of their scholastic performance as judged by their rank in class. Height and weight as well as medical and surgical illness and principal acquisitions such as walking, speech and scholastic performance did not show pathological features.

A retrospective study by Wennerholm et al. showed similar results regarding postnatal growth and health development (Wennerholm et al. 1998). A group of 255 children conceived from cryopreserved embryos were compared with 255 infants born after IVF with fresh embryos and with 252 spontaneously conceived children. The examination period covered the first 18 months. Matching was done for maternal age, parity, single/twin pregnancies and date of delivery.

Table 8.3. Perinatal outcome and follow-up of children born from cryopreserved embryos

Study	Cryopreservation group (no. of children)	Control group		Age of children (months)	Tests	Results
		No. of children				
Sutcliffe et al. 1995b	91	83	Spontaneously conceived	25 cryopreservation, 29 control	Griffith Scales	No difference
Olivennes et al. 1996	89			12–108	Physical development/ scholastic performance	No difference
Wenner- holm et al. 1998	255	255	Fresh IVF	First 18	Standard Swedish growth charts	No difference
		252	Spontaneously conceived			

Application of standard Swedish growth charts demonstrated similar postnatal growth and development in all three groups. Furthermore, there were no differences in the prevalence of chronic diseases among the three groups.

A summary of these data is presented in Table 8.3.

Conclusion

The development of children born after ART procedures was followed up in several studies in the 1980s and 1990s. Some of these studies, however, were not performed prospectively, and some others did not include a control group. Therefore, the information on this topic – despite a lot of children included – is still not optimal. However, evaluation of the data available suggests that parents can be counselled that their children will develop normally up to 10 years of age and more. This seems to be independent of the technique of ART used or the use of cryopreservation before a transfer.

9 Development of Children of Lesbian Mothers After Using Assisted Reproduction Techniques

Constanze Banz, Michael Ludwig

During recent years there have been many changes in patterns of family life (Rutter et al. 1970). More couples are living together without getting married. The proportion of children born outside marriage has risen. A lot of women with small children go out to work, so more preschool children experience some form of group day-care. The divorce rate has risen several times and many more children are being brought up in single-parent households. So the historically "most favourable" home environment provided by the middle-class, two-parent family, in which the father is paid to work outside the home and mother is not, is no longer standard.

However, even if this development is accepted, there is still a difference between those couples having a heterosexual and those having a homosexual relationship. Heterosexuality is generally accepted as being more "natural" than homosexuality. Since particularly lesbian couples not rarely have the wish for a child, the question has risen as to whether these couples should be treated using assisted reproductive techniques (ART). A special point here is not whether a single doctor takes responsibility for the treatment of these couples but whether there are any differences in the development of the children born in those relationships. Therefore, we need to examine evidence from the social sciences regarding the personal and social development of children conceived after using ART by lesbian women.

Development of Children of Lesbian Mothers in General

Systematic research seeking differences between children who have grown up with lesbian and non-lesbian mothers has taken place over the last 25 years. The preponderance of research to date has focused on children who were born in the context of heterosexual marriages, whose parents have divorced, and whose mothers have identified themselves as lesbian. It has been widely believed that children living in families headed by divorced but heterosexual mothers provide the best comparison group. Research studies on sexual identity, personal development and social relationships among these children have been carried out.

Sexual identity consists of three aspects:

- gender identity: a person's self-identification as male or female
- gender-role behaviour: the extent to which a person's activities, occupations and the like, are regarded by the culture as masculine, feminine or both
- sexual orientation: a person's choice of sexual partner

All three aspects of sexual identity have been addressed in several studies.

Gender Identity

Kirkpatrick et al. compared 20 children aged 5–12 years of lesbian mothers with 20 same-age children of single heterosexual mothers by projecting testing (Kirkpatrick et al. 1981). Of the children in each group, 16 drew a same-sex figure first, a finding within expected norms. Only three of the eight children – one girl with a lesbian mother and two boys with a heterosexual mother – who drew an opposite-sex figure first, showed concern about gender issues in clinical interviews. Golombok et al. studied gender identity among 37 children of lesbian mothers at the ages of 5 to 17 years and 38 same-age children of single heterosexual mothers by interviewing the mothers and the children. All children were happy with the sex to which they belonged and had no wish to be a member of the opposite sex (Golombok et al. 1983) (Table 9.1).

Gender Role Behaviour

A number of studies have examined gender role behaviour among children of lesbian mothers and single heterosexual mothers. In 1978 Green et al. asked 21 children of lesbian mothers which was their favourite toy (Green 1978). Of the 21 children, 20 reported a toy consistent with "conventional sex-typed preferences" as described by Green in a previous article (Green 1974). All children reported vocational choices within typical limits for conventional sex roles. Hoeffer et al. also reported no significant differences in toy choices or activity preferences among children aged 6–9 years of lesbian and single heterosexual mothers (Hoeffer 1981), 20 children in each group. Most mothers in this study said that

Table 9.1. Children's friendships differentiated according to their mothers sexual orientation (Golombok et al. 1983)

Friends	Boys		Girls	
	Lesbian mother	Single mother	Lesbian mother	Single mother
Mainly same sex	5	13	8	2
Mixed	3	5	8	3
Mainly opposite sex	0	1	0	0

they believed the toy and activity choices at this age were mostly influenced by the peer group of the children.

Golombok et al. 1983 assessed children's sex role behaviour in interviews with children and mothers (Golombok et al. 1983). To do this they used an adapted standardized interview previously developed to assess various aspects of personal and family functioning that showed good reliability and validity (Brown and Rutter 1966; Quinton et al. 1976). Both the lesbian and single-mother groups were obtained through advertisement and through contacts with gay and single-parent organizations. There were 27 families in each group, 37 children aged 5 to 17 years in the lesbian households (13 boys and 24 girls) and 38 in the single-mother households (24 boys and 14 girls). The children's sex role behaviour was assessed on two scales based on the interview with the mothers. On both scales, the scores of the boys and the girls in the two groups were closely similar. Green and colleagues interviewed 56 children of lesbian mothers and 48 children of heterosexual mothers (Green et al. 1986). No differences were detected with respect to favourite television programmes, television characters, games or toys between the two groups.

Rees administered the Bem Sex Role Inventory, a standardized instrument for evaluating an individual's sex role, to 12 children of lesbian mothers and 12 children of single heterosexual mothers (Rees 1979). The average age was 14 years with a range from 10 to 20 years. The groups did not differ on masculinity or on androgyny. Finally, Gottman et al. compared 35 adult daughters of lesbian mothers with 35 daughters of divorced and remarried heterosexual mothers and 35 daughters of single heterosexual mothers (Gottman 1990). They reported no significant differences in gender role preferences of the woman in the three groups.

Sexual Orientation

In studies of other aspects of personality and development among children of lesbian mothers, a broad array of characteristics have been assessed. In summary – as shown by the studies cited below – concerns about difficulties in personal development are not sustained by the results of existing research.

Golombok et al. collected ratings of children on a wide array of behavioural and emotional problems (Golombok et al. 1983). Gottman examined personality characteristics among adult daughters of lesbian and heterosexual mothers (Gottman 1990). Puryear studied self-concepts of children of lesbian mothers (Puryear 1983). Rees examined the development of moral judgement among teenage offspring of lesbian and heterosexual mothers (Rees 1979). Green assessed intelligence among children of these two groups (Green et al. 1986). No significant differences could be found in these studies, which are outlined below.

Golombok et al. assessed the heterosexual versus homosexual interests of older children (Golombok et al. 1983). There were 9 children of lesbian mothers and 11 of heterosexual mothers. The precise ages of the children were not reported. Among the nine children in the lesbian households, six showed a definite heterosexual interest, two exhibited no particular interest in either direction and one girl had a homosexual interest. In the single-mother group, seven had not yet shown a definite sexual interest and the remaining four exhibited a clearly heterosexual interest. No lesbian mother expressed a clear preference for homosexuality and none wished to influence their children in this direction.

Huggins (1989) interviewed 36 boys and girls between 13 and 19 years, 18 of lesbian mothers and 18 of heterosexual mothers. No child of a lesbian mother and one child of a heterosexual mother was identified as homosexual. This difference was not statistically significant (Huggins 1989). In a study by Gottman, 16% of daughters of lesbian and heterosexual mothers self-identified as lesbians (Gottman 1990). The percentages of lesbian daughters did not vary as a function of their mother's sexual orientation.

Other Aspects of Personality Development

Overall development of gender identity, of gender role behaviour and of sexual preference among offspring of lesbian mothers was found to fall within normal bounds in each study. However, one has to take into consideration that most of the studies assessed children, but many homosexual people do not self-identify as homosexual until adulthood. Therefore, a final judgement regarding this question cannot be made.

In studies of other aspects of personal development among children of lesbian mothers, a broad array of characteristics, such as separation-individuation, psychiatric evaluation, behaviour problems, personality, self-concept, locus of control, moral judgement and intelligence, have been assessed. Golombok et al. assessed behavioural problems of children using parents' and teachers' questionnaires (Golombok et al. 1983). The teachers did not know the sexual orientation of the mothers. The proportion of children scoring above a cut-off point tended to be higher in the single-parent group, but not significantly: 33.3% of sons and 16.6% of daughters of lesbian mothers, and 36.3% of sons and 28.5% of daughters of heterosexual mothers on the teachers scale.

Puryear studied self-concepts among 15 elementary school children of lesbians and 15 children of heterosexual woman, and found that their self-concepts were within the normal range in both groups (Puryear 1983). Rees assessed the moral maturity between the children of lesbian versus heterosexual mothers (Rees 1979). Using techniques developed by Kohlberg (Kohlberg 1964), maturity of moral judgement in this study was assessed using the adolescents' responses to hypothetical moral dilemmas. There were no differences between the two groups. Green and colleagues used a standardized individual test of intelligence for two groups of children (Green et al. 1986). There were no differences in intelligence between children of lesbian and heterosexual mothers.

In summary, fears that children of lesbian mothers suffer deficits in personal development are without empirical foundation, although most of theses studies investigated only small numbers of children in the assessed groups.

Children's Social Relationships

Some studies assessing potential differences between children of homosexual versus heterosexual mothers have included assessments of the children's social relationships. Green interviewed 21 elementary school children of lesbian mothers concerning their friends (Green 1978). A predominantly same-sex peer group of friends were named by 19 of the children. The result was considered to be normal for this age group. In the study by Golombok et al. most children of lesbian and heterosexual mothers named a predominantly same-sex peer group (Golombok et al. 1983). There were no significant differences between the two groups (Table 9.1).

Kirkpatrick et al. investigated children's contact with adult men in lesbian mother versus heterosexual mothers homes (Kirkpatrick et al. 1981). Interestingly they reported that lesbian mothers were more concerned that their children have opportunities for good relationships with adult men. Kirkpatrick even indicated that lesbian mothers had more adult male family friends than heterosexual single mothers (Kirkpatrick 1987). Golombok et al. assessed children's relationships with their fathers (Golombok et al. 1983). Of 37 children of lesbian mothers, 12 were reported as having contact with their fathers at least once a week, but only 2 of 38 children of single heterosexual mothers. Of 38 children of heterosexual mothers, 22 (57.9%) had had no contact with their fathers during the last year, but only 15 of 37 children (40.5%) of lesbian mothers, which is a significant difference ($P < 0.05$). In summary, most children of lesbian mothers had at least some contact with their fathers, whereas most children of heterosexual mothers did not.

Harris and Turner studied homosexual and heterosexual parents (Harris and Turner 1985). A significant difference between the two groups was that heterosexual parents were more likely to mention that their children's visits with the other parent presented problems for them.

There are concerns that children of homosexual parents are more likely to be sexually abused than children of heterosexual parents. Results of research in this area show that the great majority of adults who perpetrate sexual abuse are male. Sexual abuse of children by adult woman is extremely rare (Finkelhor and Russell 1984; Jones and MacFarlane 1980; Sarafino 1979). The overwhelming majority of cases concerning sexual abuse of a child can be characterized as "heterosexual" with an adult male abusing a young female. Therefore, this concern does not have any fundamental basis in the literature.

Tasker and Golombok reported a special study in 1995, in which they performed a further follow-up of the children and mothers whom they had already interviewed for a previous study (Tasker and Golombok 1995). In the initial study, the average age of the children was 9.5 years. In the follow-up study the average age was 23.5 years (range 17–35 years). Only 62% of the children were able to be interviewed between 1991 and 1992: 8 sons and 17 daughters of a lesbian mother, and 12 sons and 9 daughters of a single heterosexual mother. Children who were aware of their mother's lesbian identity at the time of the original study in 1983 tended to be more likely to participate in the follow-up study.

To describe family relationships, most young adults from both types of family background were able to report on their experience of step-family relationships. Young adults who had been brought up in a lesbian household described their relationship with their mother's partner more positively ($P < 0.01$) than did those who had been raised by a heterosexual mother and her new partner. In adulthood young adults brought up by a lesbian mother were significantly ($P < 0.05$) more positive about their mother's non-conventional relationships and were more likely to be proud of their mother's sexual identity than were those raised by a single heterosexual mother.

Young adults from a lesbian family were no more likely to remember general teasing by their peers than were those from a heterosexual single-parent home. With respect to teasing about their sexuality, those from a lesbian family were more likely to recall having been teased about being gay or lesbian themselves.

No significant difference was found between young adults from lesbian and heterosexual single mothers who had experienced sexual orientation through someone of the same gender (9/25 versus 4/20). However, five daughters and one son of a lesbian mother who reported same-gender sexual attraction, had also been involved in a same-gender sexual relationship, whereas none of the children of a heterosexual mother who reported same-gender attraction had done so. Furthermore, young adults with a lesbian mother were significantly ($p < 0.003$) more likely to report having considered the possibility of becoming involved in a same-gender sexual relationship.

To check psychological well-being, the Trait Anxiety Inventory (Spielberger 1983) and the Beck Depression Inventory (Beck and Steer 1987) were applied. There were no significant differences between young adults from lesbian or heterosexual mothers in terms of anxiety and depression. A similar proportion of participants from both groups reported contact with health-care professionals for problems with anxiety, depression or stress.

Children Conceived Via Donor Insemination by Lesbian Mothers

In many countries, for example Germany, ART is generally not offered to lesbian women. It is argued that a lesbian mother, eventually with her partner, is not an adequate substitute for the "traditional" family for a child and may impair the child's well-being.

In some countries that view has changed. The example of New Zealand shows this development in law. In 1977 the Human Rights Commission Act passed which makes discrimination unlawful on the grounds of race, colour, ethic or national origins, sex, religion and marital status (New Zealand Government 1977). In 1993 these grounds were extended to include disability, sexual orientation and family status (New Zealand Government 1993). The Status of Children Amendment Act 1987 (New Zealand Government 1987) established, that in cases where third party gametes were used in ART the legal father of the resulting offspring is the consenting partner of the woman undergoing the treatment. This legislation removes the possibility that the donor could be required to provide child support or could gain access to the offspring. Since 1994 it is a contravention of the Human Rights Act to refuse lesbian woman access to ART, and therefore it is illegal in New Zealand (New Zealand Government 1993). On the other hand, health professionals are allowed a conscience clause as is the case in abortion, which allows them to refuse to administer certain services as long as they refer patients to someone who will provide this service. In addition, lesbian women may have to pay full cost for their treatment while medically infertile couples are subsidized by the state.

Lesbian women are normally able to have offspring if they were to undertake sexual intercourse with a fertile man. They are fertile individuals. They may be considered to be "socially" infertile in that for most of them to have sexual intercourse with a man in order to have a child would be counter to their sexual orientation or to their morality. So most of the lesbian women who want to become pregnant ask for donor insemination (AID). There are even negative consequences associated with denying lesbian woman access to AID. They may resort to insemination using either known donors or anonymous donors accessed through a go-between. This places these women at a greater risk of contracting genetic diseases and sexually transmitted diseases such as HIV. As we know in the abortion situation health professionals do not prevent abortion by denying doing it.

But what about the main argument in this discussion: do children conceived via AID and who grow up with a lesbian mother have any special problems? First, the data mentioned above on children with lesbian mothers, are clearly against this.

However, there are mainly two studies that investigated exactly this field. The first by Brewaeys et al. was published in 1997. A total of 30 lesbian mother families (LeDI) with children aged 4–8 years resulting from AID were compared with 38 heterosexual families with a child resulting from AID (HeDI) and with 30 heterosexual families (NC) who had naturally conceived a child. All lesbian families, where the mother had attended the Fertility Department of the Brussels University Hospital between 1986 and 1991 for AID, were asked to take part in the study. The response rate was 100%. This study sample may therefore be considered to be truly representative of the general population of lesbian mothers who attend a fertility clinic in order to conceive. The control groups were recruited through the University Hospital Leiden. The response rates were 53% for HeDI families and 60% for the NC families. Both parents were asked to take part in the interview, which took place at home. For lesbian mother families, 28 of the 30 interviews involved both mothers, for HeDI families 29 out of 38 fathers were involved and for NC families 15 out of 30 fathers took part in the interview.

No significant differences were found between the groups for the mean age of the children, mean age of the biological mother and mean age of the social mother or the father. The number of children in the family did not differ among the groups. Significant differences between groups were found for the educational level. Heterosexual AID parents had a lower educational level than lesbian mothers or NC parents.

A significant difference was found for the quality of the parent-child inter-action which was higher for the lesbian social mothers than for the heterosexual fathers ($P < 0.001$). The quality of parent-child interaction was assessed accord-ing to the parent's report of the time spent together with the child, their enjoy-ment of each other's company, their play activities and their expressed physical affection for each other. Among the lesbian mothers, the quality of the parent-child interaction did not differ between the biological mother and the social mother. Significantly more ($P < 0.001$) lesbian mothers (58%) had a full-time job than did the HeDI mothers (24%) or NC mothers (9%). Most of the LeDI social mothers (86%) worked full-time, equivalent to 94% of the HeDI fathers and 86% of the NC fathers. But social mothers of lesbian families were signifi-cantly more involved in practical childcare activities compared with fathers in the two heterosexual groups, while AID fathers were more active ($P < 0.05$) in helping their partners than were NC fathers. Equal sharing occurred in 50% of the lesbian mother families and in none of the heterosexual families. Social mothers of lesbian families even helped their partners significantly more often ($P < 0.05$) in disciplining the child than did fathers in the two control groups.

All children from lesbian mother families reported not having a father and chose both biological and social mother as family members. All children except one were informed about their mothers having used a donor for insemination. Of the heterosexual parents only one couple had already told and eight wanted to tell later. Comparing the total problem scores of the study groups with those of a Dutch population sample, significant differences were found for the hetero-sexual AID families, with children having higher total problem scores. No dif-ferences were found in terms of the children's gender or the parent's education-al level.

The second very important study in this area is that by Chan et al. (1998). The authors contacted 108 families who were clients of The Sperm Bank California and conceived and gave birth to children prior to July 1990. Families headed by lesbian mothers and by couples were more likely ($P < 0.05$) to have been suc-cessfully contacted than were those headed by heterosexual or single parents. Of 80 families who agreed to participate in the research, 55 were headed by a les-bian, 25 by a heterosexual, and 50 by couples and 30 by single mothers. Children averaged 7 years of age and biological mothers averaged 42 years of age. There was no difference in mothers' or children's' age between the different groups. The family incomes were well above the national average. Besides a higher educa-tional level of the lesbian mothers, no significant demographic differences among the four family types were found. The participating families completed several tests such as the Child Behaviour Checklist (Achenbach 1991a), the Teacher Report Form (Achenbach 1991b), the Parenting Stress Index-Short Form (Abidin 1995) and the Locke-Wallace Marital Adjustment Test (Locke and Wallace 1959).

The results showed no significant differences in child adjustment as a func-tion of parental sexual orientation or number of parents at home. Children's behavioural problems as reported by parents were significantly correlated with the parents' own adjustment. When parents reported more parenting distress and more dysfunctional parent-child interactions, children exhibited more behaviour problems. Parents' sexual orientation and relationship status were unrelated to children's behaviour problems as reported by the biological mother. Nonbiological parents' reports of dysfunctional parent-child interactions were significantly associated with children's behaviour problems. Fathers tended to describe their children in more favourable terms than did mothers. Among families headed by couples, better relationship adjustment within the couples was associated with fewer behaviour problems among the children. Conflict between parents was associated with difficulties in child adjustment.

In summary, among families headed by heterosexual or homosexual couples, children were rated as better adjusted when their parents reported greater relationship satisfaction, higher levels of love and lower interparental conflict.

Conclusion

There is no evidence to suggest that development of children of lesbian mothers conceived via AID is compromised in any respect relative to that of offspring of heterosexual single mothers or heterosexual parents after AID. Despite long-standing legal presumptions against lesbian mothers in many states, not a single study has found children of lesbian mothers to be disadvantaged in any significant respect relative to children of heterosexual mothers or parents after AID. Children of lesbian mothers conceived via AID grow up in a warm and secure family environment. The social mothers show great interaction with the children. Furthermore, these families are at least as open to other persons – male and female – as compared to the traditional "mother-father-child" family.

Therefore, one has to realize, that the question regarding child outcome in those families results more from traditional ideas about sexual orientation than from facts. The studies clearly prove, that children's well-being is more a function of parenting and the relationship process within the family than a function of household composition or demographic factors. Child behaviour problems are best understood as the result of interparental conflict rather than the parental sexual orientation or family structure.

To conclude, a prohibition of ART procedures in female homosexual relationships cannot be justified on the basis of different development of children during their first years of life or a "worse" family quality.

10 Development of Children and Family Structure After IVF and Gamete Donation

Constanze Banz, Michael Ludwig

The creation of families by means of reproductive technologies has raised important questions about the development of the children, the well-being of the children, the relationship of the child with its environment, and the consequences for the parent-child relationship, particularly where gamete donation has been used to conceive the child. It has been suggested that couples who have not come to terms with their infertility may experience difficulties in the relationship with their child. After donor insemination (AID) the child is genetically related to the mother but not to the father, which may theoretically lead to further problems in either the father-child or child-father relationship.

Children and Their Parents After IVF

A study by Stanton and Golombok published in 1993 examined the degree of anxiety experienced by pregnant women who had conceived by IVF, their attitudes towards the pregnancy and the strength of their attachment to the fetus (Golombok et al. 1993). The strength of maternal-fetal attachment increases as pregnancy progresses, with the perception of fetal movement marking an important stage in the development of maternal feelings. Ultrasound scanning has also been found to increase the mother's feelings towards the fetus. In this study, 15 women who had conceived by IVF were compared with 20 woman who had conceived without assistance. All of the pregnant woman were recruited from King's Hospital in London and had reached at least 20 weeks of gestation. The response rate was 100%. The 15 woman who had conceived after IVF were randomly selected. The average age was 34 years and the average length of gestation was 31 weeks. All had taken over a year to conceive, the majority over 5 years; 13 were primiparous. The average age of the woman with naturally conceived pregnancies was 30 years and the average length of gestation was 34 weeks. None had taken longer than 1 year to conceive and 19 were expecting their first child. Woman were asked to complete the State-Trait Anxiety Inventory (Spielberger 1983) which provides a separate score for state and trait anxiety, the Maternal-Fetal Attachment Scale (MFAS) (Cranley 1981) which produces an overall score of strength of attachment to the fetus, and the Childbearing Attitudes questionnaire (CAQ) (Ruble et al. 1990). No statistically significant differences between the groups were found for state or trait anxiety. Women with an IVF pregnancy were equally attached to their fetus. But women who had conceived by IVF obtained significantly lower scores than women in the control group on the CAQ ($P < 0.01$), reflecting a poorer relationship with their husband and greater social boredom.

In contrast to these results, other studies have shown very low rates of divorce or separation for IVF couples. In a detailed examination of the relationship between the MFAS and the CAQ, correlations were found to be statistically significant for the interaction with the fetus ($P < 0.01$) and role-taking. In both groups, less-positive attitudes towards childbearing were associated with weaker attachment behaviour such as talking to the fetus and imagining what it would be like to look after the baby. The women who had conceived by IVF did not show weaker attachment to their fetus or more negative attitudes towards childbearing.

Raoul-Duval et al. were the first to perform a psychological follow-up of children born after IVF (Raoul-Duval et al. 1994). The study comprised 33 children conceived by IVF, 33 children conceived naturally and 14 children born after oocyte donation seen after delivery, and at 9 months, 18 months and 3 years. All children were born between 1987 and 1989 at term as singletons. Parents were volunteers who were involved in a semidirective interview and answered a questionnaire. In the post-partum period there were slightly more mother-infant communication problems in the IVF group than in the other two groups. Slightly more of these women showed signs of depression. The proportion of women who decided to breast-feed was similar in the three groups. At 9 months sleep disorders were more frequent in the infants in the IVF group, and mothers after IVF still showed more signs of depression of the neurotic type. The infants' sleep disorders often corresponded to maternal problems and usually disappeared when the mother's state improved. None of the mothers or their children required treatment for these disorders. Five of the woman in the IVF group became pregnant again, compared to none in the control group and one in the oocyte donation group. At 18 months the differences were less marked, and at 36 months the incidence of sleep disorders was similar in the three groups of children and there was further decrease in the frequency of depression in the IVF group. The ovum donation programme showed an excellent mother-infant relationship and problem-free pregnancies.

The cognitive, behavioural and social development (see Chapter 8) of children born after IVF was assessed in a study by Cederblad et al. (1996). Included in the study were 99 children, 52 girls and 47 boys born between 1983 and 1991 in Malmö after IVF; 27 (27.3%) children were born prematurely. Mothers were interviewed by a trained child psychologist. Children were assessed using the Griffith developmental scale (Griffith 1970), which measures the locomotor scale, the personal social scale, hearing and speech scale, eye and hand co-ordination scale, performance scale and the logic scale. The interview covered 50 different behaviours and psychosomatic symptoms. The mean age of the children was 62 months (range 33–85 months). The average age of the mothers at the time of birth was 33 years (range 26–41 years) and of the fathers 35 years (range 26–47 years). At the time of birth all couples were married or cohabiting and 92% were still married or cohabiting at the time of the study. The data were

Table 10.1. Percentage of IVF children behaviourally disturbed compared to a control population (Cederblad et al. 1996)

	IVF (%)	Control group (%)
All children	6	13
2–4 years	0	16
5–7 years	9	11

compared with those of a Swedish epidemiological study of 345 subjects investigated with the same techniques and were the same age group as in the study group (Cederblad and Höök 1991). The percentage of children above the cut-off score for disturbed behaviour did not differ between the IVF children and the control group (Table 10.1). In the youngest age group (2–4 years), the IVF group was less disturbed than the control children. Both sexes showed the same pattern. The IVF families were very happy to have a child. They showed strong, positive interest in the child. The children were engaged in many activities both together with the parents and in activities with other children outside the home. In conclusion the investigation showed that the intellectual, emotional, somatic and social development of the children born after IVF was very satisfactory.

A first interim analysis of The European Study of assisted reproduction families by Golombok et al. was published in 1996 (Golombok et al. 1996). Two northern European countries (UK and the Netherlands) and two southern European countries (Spain and Italy) participated in the study. Recruited into the study by infertility clinics were 116 families with a child conceived by IVF and 111 families with a child conceived by AID. Control groups of 115 adoptive families and 120 families with a naturally conceived child were also included. Children were aged 4–8 years. Children with major congenital abnormalities or children who had experienced perinatal complications and children of multiple birth were not included in the study. In each country there were similar proportions of boys and girls in each group. Although complete matching was not achieved, the group and country differences that were identified for the age of the child and the mother, and for social class and family size, were not relevant. Data were collected from both parents by questionnaires and additionally from the mother by interview. The children's' teachers also completed questionnaires. Parents completed the Golombok Rust Inventory of Marital State (Rust et al. 1988), the Trait Anxiety Inventory (Spielberger 1983) and the Beck Depression Inventory (Beck and Steer 1987). The quality of parenting was assessed by standardized interview with the mother using an adaptation of the technique developed by Quinton and Rutter (1988). The presence of behavioural or emotional problems in the children was assessed using the Rutter 'A' scale completed by the child's mother, and the Rutter 'B' scale completed by the child's teacher (Rutter et al. 1970). A modified version of the Family Relations Test (Bene and Anthony 1985) was administered to the children to obtain a standardized assessment of the children's feeling about their parents. The Pictorial Scale of Perceived Competence and Social Acceptance for Young Children (Harter and Pike 1984) was also administered to each child.

Almost all of the parents were married. Only 15 couples (3.3%) had separated or divorced (seven IVF, two AID, one adoptive and five natural conception). The quality of the parents' relationship indicated a lower incidence of marital difficulties among adoptive mothers ($P < 0.001$) but not for fathers. A significant difference in anxiety level as assessed by the Trait Anxiety Inventory was found for mothers ($P < 0.05$) but not for fathers, reflecting lower anxiety levels among mothers with an assisted reproduction child than among mothers with a naturally conceived child ($P < 0.01$). The Beck Depression Inventory showed lower levels of depression among assisted reproduction mothers than among mothers with a naturally conceived child ($P < 0.05$). Mothers with a child conceived by assisted reproduction expressed significantly greater warmth towards their child than mothers with a naturally conceived child ($P < 0.001$). There was no significant difference between adoptive mothers, IVF mothers and AID mothers. Mothers of a child conceived by assisted reproduction showed greater emotional involvement with their child ($P < 0.001$). Fathers of children conceived by assisted reproduction showed greater interaction with their children ($P < 0.01$). There was no significant difference between IVF, AID and adoptive fathers. Spanish AID fathers reported less parenting stress than fathers from other countries and more parenting stress was reported by adoptive fathers in Italy ($P < 0.05$). Assisted reproduction fathers were more involved in care-giving than fathers of naturally conceived children ($P < 0.01$). Children did not differ with respect to the presence of emotional or behavioural problems. The teachers' ratings of the children's' emotional and behavioural difficulties also did not differ according to family type.

This study is certainly of outstanding importance due to its size and controlled design. The findings have a high value and are quite reliable, especially since they have been confirmed by other, smaller, studies, which are also discussed in this chapter.

Another study investigated parental stress and child behaviour in families with twins conceived by IVF (Cook et al. 1998). A total of 12 families with twins conceived by IVF were approached through UK fertility clinics. A control group of 14 with naturally conceived twins was recruited. There was no significant difference between the proportion of boys and girls in each group. The procedure of the study was the same as in the study discussed above (Golombok et al. 1996). There were no significant differences between groups for mother's warmth or emotional involvement, but parents of IVF twins reported significantly higher levels of stress than parents of naturally conceived children ($P < 0.01$). Fathers of IVF twins reported their interactions with their children to be less rewarding, and the children themselves more difficult to deal with ($P < 0.01$). No significant differences were found on these subscales for mothers. None of the children had scores indicating the presence of psychiatric disorder.

A French study by Garel and Bondel published in 1992 assessed the psychological consequences for mothers of having triplets 1 year after birth (Garel and Blondel 1992). Home visits were made to 12 mothers of triplets 1 year after the birth. Tape-recorded semistructured interviews were conducted by a psychologist. All mothers except one were primiparae. One pregnancy was spontaneous, 11 had been initiated after ovarian stimulation (two women) or in vitro fertilization or gamete intrafallopian transfer (nine women). In most of the cases, home help was no longer provided by the social services and half of the fathers had stopped helping their wife. The few mothers who were still extensively helped at 1 year mentioned fewer physical and psychological troubles. A majority of mothers suffered from isolation. They were seldom able to go out of the house for their own needs or social activities without the children. Most mothers reported difficulties with their marital relationship. One husband had left home.

Mothers often said it was difficult for them to give adequate attention to the three children and mentioned feelings of exasperation or hostility towards the children. It is also interesting to note that mothers tended to give special treatment to one of the children – either in a positive or a negative sense. This may have been due to the fact that twins are the maximum number of children that can have the mother's full attention. Therefore, in the case of triplets, the mother cannot give adequate attention to all the children. Three mothers were treated for major depressive disorders, six others experienced serious psychological difficulties such as asthenia, anxiety and helplessness. A follow-up of these families 7 years after birth (Garel et al. 2001) showed an improvement in the situation, but the mother's psychological distress and quality of relationship with the children remained a preoccupation in 50%.

These results suggest that families with twins or higher-order births should not be excluded from studies of the psychological consequences of assisted reproduction. They are in particular need of support.

Children and Their Parents After Gamete Donation

One of the first pilot studies dealing with family structure following donor insemination was by Clayton and Kovacs (1982). In this study, 50 couples were interviewed by a social worker in the presence of the child conceived by AID. The age of the children was between 12 and 36 months. The type of interview is not described further. All wives were anxious about their husband's reaction to the child, but only four (8%) admitted having any problems. One husband felt that the child was a constant reminder of his infertility. Of the 50 couples, 34 (68%) stated they would not tell the child about his or her origin; 7 thought they would explain, and 9 were unsure. Further AID children were definitely wanted by 40 couples, and 18 mothers had already conceived again.

Amuzu et al. evaluated the pregnancies of 357 woman who conceived through AID between 1976 and 1988 (Amuzu et al. 1990). Initial phone contact was followed by a postal questionnaire. They determined the status of the marriage and attitudes about confidentiality concerning the origins of their children. The indications for AID included azoospermia (31%), oligospermia (35%), and vasectomy (21%). Most of the families had one AID child, whereas 31% had two or more, and the largest family had five children through AID. Only one couple (0.3 %) had already informed their child of its origin; 47 % said they would not, 13 % said they would eventually and 40 % remained undecided. Of the respondents, 54 % thought that AID had improved their marriage, whereas 3 % thought it had had a detrimental effect. All of the respondents were women. The divorce rate was 7.2 % and was significantly lower ($P < 0.01$) among the couples with AID children than the expected rate of 12.9 % for an age-matched group followed over the same period.

Daniels reported a study addressing the question as to why couples decide to seek AID instead of adoption (Daniels 1994). Interviews were conducted with 58 couples with a child conceived by AID between 1984 and 1990. Each partner separately completed a questionnaire. The interviews covered such aspects as the couple's relationship, adoption, attitudes towards AID, and relationship with the child. Of the 58 couples, 72 % had thought about adoption or had made some approach towards adoption, 33 % had only thought about it, and 22 % had begun an adoption procedure but 33 % of these had had such a negative experience that they gave up. AID was viewed as the preferred option mainly because it gave the female partner the opportunity to be pregnant and experience giving birth. The ease of obtaining a child via AID was given as a reason for choosing AID by 47 %. The biological-ethical linkage was seen to be an advantage by only 21% of the couples.

Although it has been suggested that secrets are detrimental to a family because they create boundaries between those who know and those who do not, most of the parents with a child conceived by AID do not tell their child about its origin. Even in Sweden, where by law a child has to be told about its origin, only 11 % of parents in a recent survey had told their child about AID, but additionally 48 % intended to tell (Gottlieb et al. 2000). Cook et al. investigated the reasons for this behaviour (Cook et al. 1995). Included in this study were 45 families with a child conceived by AID and two comparison groups, one of 55 families with a child adopted at or shortly after birth, and 41 families with a child conceived by IVF. The children were between 4 and 8 years of age. Families who had twins or children from a higher-order multiple birth or with a major congenital abnormality or had experienced perinatal complications were excluded. The proportion of boys and girls in each group of families was similar. None of the AID parents had told their children about the method of their conception. This contrasts sharply with the adoption group, where children in all but one family (98 %) had been told. In the IVF group, 11 couples (26.8 %) had already told their children, 22 (53.6 %) planned to tell, 5 (12.2 %) were unsure, and 3 (7.3 %) had decided not to tell. Towards family members there was different behaviour. Of the AID parents, 50 % had told one family member. All the adoptive parents had told someone, and 93 % of the IVF parents had done so. Of the AID mothers who reported that they had decided not to tell, 70 % had made this decision in order to protect their child. Only two of the IVF mothers and none of the adoptive parents gave this reason. Protecting the father was a concern of 69 % of the AID parents. First they were afraid that the child would not love the father any more, and second that other people would learn about the father's infertility.

Even those AID parents who intended to tell had not made plans about when or how to do so. There was no consensus about the appropriate age to tell. These issues did not present such a problem for adoptive parents – all but one couple had already told. However, adoptive parents reported that they had been advised by social workers or social services to tell their children. None of the IVF and only two of the AID parents reported that they received any advice from the clinic. AID parents were also often conscious of the difficulty of providing information about the donor, because mostly they knew nearly nothing about him.

These data show the sharp contrast between disclosure towards the child and discussing the subject of AID with family members or friends in 50%. It creates a problematic situation, since it cannot be guaranteed that the child will not learn about its origin. In certain situations it might happen that a third person will tell the child, which might lead to severe problems in the parent-child relationship. Therefore, telling a third person about a child's origin instead of telling the child directly is the real problem.

A further study by Golombok et al. compared children's socioemotional development and the family structure of children conceived by oocyte or sperm donation (Golombok et al. 1999). Recruited into the study were 41 families with a child conceived by IVF, 45 families with a child conceived by AID and 21 families with a child conceived by oocyte donation. IVF and AID children were between 4 and 8 years old, and the oocyte donation children had the lower age limit of 3.5 years. The donor was anonymous to all of the AID families and to 18 (85.7%) of the oocyte donation families. There were similar proportions of boys and girls in each group of families. Data were collected from the mother by interview, from both parents by questionnaire, and from the child using a standardized test.

The mothers of genetically unrelated children reported greater marital satisfaction than mothers of genetically related children ($P < 0.05$) irrespective of whether or not the father had a genetic link with the child. They reported lower levels of parenting stress when the child had a genetic link with the father ($P < 0.01$). Fathers showed lower levels of stress when the child was genetically unrelated to the mother ($P < 0.01$) whether or not there was a genetic link with the father. A significant difference was found between groups for warmth, with less warmth for the child expressed by mothers ($P < 0.05$) when the child was not genetically related to the father irrespective of whether or not there was a genetic link with the mother. The children's socioemotional development showed no significant main effect for genetic relatedness to the mother. In families where the child was not genetically related to the mother but had a genetic link with the father, mothers reported lower levels of parental distress and more coordination with the father over discipline of the child. These feelings of security seem to lead to greater warmth for the child.

There was a significant difference ($P < 0.05$) for cognitive competence, showing that children who were genetically unrelated to their father perceived themselves to be more cognitively competent than children who shared a genetic link with their father whether or not they were genetically related to their mother. This finding might, as discussed by the authors, reflect a real difference in cognitive competence, because a high proportion of sperm donors are students, and many are medical students (Cook et al. 1995).

None of the parents with a child conceived by AID, and only one of the oocyte donation parents had told their child about the method of conception. Parents who planned never to tell their child – 82% of the AID parents and 38% of the oocyte donation parents – or were undecided on this issue were asked to give their reasons. Of the AID parents and the oocyte donation parents, 49% and 69%, respectively, wished to protect the child. The wish to protect the mother was given as a reason by 19% of the AID parents and 23% of the oocyte donation parents. The wish to protect the child was given by 69% of the AID parents and 23% of the oocyte donation parents. Surprisingly, 85% of the AID parents and 69% of the oocyte donation parents felt that there was no need to tell the child.

Turner and Coyle tried to answer the question as to what it means for a child to be the offspring of gamete donation (Turner and Coyle 2000). After contacting donor conception support networks, 16 adults contacted the researchers voluntarily and answered a semistructured questionnaire. There were 13 female and 3 male participants, with a mean age of 44.6 years (range 26–55 years). Most of them were born and lived in the USA. Many participants reported feeling shocked at discovering their status as donor offspring, and that the safety of their familiar world had been lost. They reported difficulties in assimilating this information. Many believed that the withholding of information about the manner of their conception had been damaging. They mistrusted the world around. The right to know their genetic origin seemed to be a common theme with all but one of the participants. Others expressed a feeling of loss not only in terms of needing to know their biological father but also in terms of feelings of being part of an unemotional procedure. Often they felt a need to search and have information about the donor and found it difficult to talk about this problem. They reported a sense of loss and grief about never being able to know their biological origin. Even though this study gives an interesting insight into this problem, one has to be aware that there must have been an enormous selection bias among the participants. It may be that those who participated in the survey were preferentially those who really had problems dealing with the information. However, the study clearly shows that there is a need to clarify when and how it is best to tell children about their origin.

Conclusion

The families created by parents and their children conceived by IVF are as normal as families arising from spontaneous conception. The mothers of these children express greater warmth towards their children, are more emotionally involved, interact more with their children and report less stress associated with parenting – as long as they are singletons – than mothers who conceived naturally. This involvement with the child starts early in pregnancy and a weaker attachment to the fetus or more negative attitudes towards childbearing is not shown. Similarly, assisted reproduction fathers are found to interact more with the child and contribute more to parenting than fathers with a naturally conceived child. With respect to the children, no overall group differences have been found in terms of the presence of psychological disorder, the children's perception of the quality of family relationships or the children's developing self-esteem. The few exceptions are almost entirely associated with the psychological state of the parents rather than with the quality of family relationships.

The consequences to parenting of twin or higher order births after assisted reproduction need further investigation, but these parents seem to need special support. It has become clear that having higher order multiples is not only a social but also a psychological catastrophe for the parents and especially for the mothers.

No significant differences have been found for the social and emotional development of children conceived by AID. The absence of a genetic relationship, in itself does not lead to difficulties for parents or children. But most of the parents of children conceived by AID do not tell their children about their origin. There are different reasons for this behaviour. Most of them claim that they want to protect the child. Some of these children feel that there is something in the family relationship that does not feel right. Most people who learn about their AID origin in adulthood report that their reaction is anger and resentment at the lies and a loss of a sense of self and of identity. All wish that they had been told much earlier and want information about the donor. In most countries the anonymity of the donor is protected by law. In the UK, however, non-identifying information from a special register can be released to the offspring when they reach the age of 18 years or in particular circumstances at 16 years.

Parents who conceived children by AID have generally not been advised to tell their children. They do not know when and how to do so. These questions as to the best time and way to tell cannot be answered by existing studies. But parents need help not only with disclosure to their children, but also with disclosure to other adults in order to obtain support.

11 General Conclusions

Michael Ludwig

The collected data in this book show that a pregnancy following ART has to be considered as a high-risk pregnancy – for several reasons.

During the first trimester there is a higher risk of ectopic and heterotopic pregnancies. Due to the different management of these pregnancies, one has also perhaps to face an increased risk of spontaneous abortion. However, since controlled studies on larger cohorts regarding this topic are not available, the only available data can be interpreted as indicating that it is the problem of infertility which increases the risk of spontaneous abortions and not the ART procedure itself.

Depending on the procedure used for ART, during the further course of pregnancy an increased risk of pregnancy complications – such as pregnancy-induced hypertension – has to be expected. This seems to be a substantial problem in IVF pregnancies, but not in others, and even not in pregnancies following ICSI. Again, this clearly shows that patients undergoing different ART procedures face a different set of potential problems. Even more, one has to expect special problems with each subgroup of these patients.

In couples suffering, for example, from male factor infertility, there are several well-defined genetic problems which are much more frequent as compared to the general fertile population. Therefore, couples undergoing ICSI are quite as indicated by, for example, very special genetic predispositions which finally lead to the treatment by ICSI: e.g. men with Kartagener syndrome have been treated by this technique successfully in the past (Cayan et al. 2001). However, it is not known how many other disturbances of sperm production and differentiation are also determined by genetic factors. Since about 30–40% of all men with eugonadotropic hypogonadism do not show any anamnestic or medical abnormality, this group may have at least one abnormal genetic factor which might also contribute to differences in abortion or malformation rates at birth.

However, intensive genetic screening showed in about 13% of 680 men undergoing ICSI the presence of certain genetic risks – chromosomal abnormalities (4.7%), CFTR mutations (0.9%), Y chromosome microdeletions (5.6%), and androgen receptor mutations (1.0%) (Foresta and Ferlin 2001). These authors were of the opinion that this could mainly explain the problem of a slightly higher risk of malformation in children born after ICSI: "congenital anomalies in ICSI children are not related to the ICSI technique, but to the seminal disorder".

An extreme example may be the successful treatment of men who suffer from Klinefelter syndrome who have also parented a couple of children in the past few years after ICSI treatment (Cruger et al. 2001). The outstanding importance of this has been shown in an in vitro FISH study of these men (Hennebicq et al. 2001). These authors studied a non-mosaic Klinefelter patient who had been accepted for inclusion in an ICSI program. Segregation analysis revealed a substantially higher rate of 24,XX (3.2%) and 24,XY (0.8%) hyperhaploid sperms as compared to two control patients (0.1 and 0.4% for 24,XX, and 0 and 0.1% for 24,XY, respectively). Furthermore, and perhaps even more importantly, there was an associated higher risk for transmission of trisomy 21 in this patient, with a higher rate of hyperhaploid sperms for chromosome 21 as compared to a control patient (6.2% versus 0.3%). This interchromosomal effect may also be true for other chromosomes, or other less apparent chromosome aberrations in infertile men as compared to a Klinefelter syndrome patient (Hennebicq et al. 2001). This is in line with the observation of a paternally induced trisomy 21 in an ICSI offspring (Bartels et al. 1998). Most gonosomal aberrations in ICSI offspring are of paternal origin (Van Opstal et al. 1997), which is not different from spontaneously conceived pregnancies.

However, these reports on the origin of abnormal karyotypes in children born after ICSI or abortion are rare. However, those that identify the mother as the origin – such as that on a monosomy 21 in abortion material – are important since they demonstrate that it is not necessarily the father who contributes to the risk (Ma et al. 2001).

The problem of infertility in relation to the outcome of pregnancies after ART has been defined by several authors. The chapter on the outcome of matched singleton pregnancies following conventional IVF as compared to spontaneously conceived singleton pregnancies illustrates very nicely that there must be additional risk factors related to infertility itself and not to the procedure. These "unknown particular negative features of the subfertile patient" (Lambalk and van Hooft 2001) have still to be identified.

In the future, there may be a greater ability to exclude genetically abnormal embryos from transfers, and thereby reduce the possibility of preclinical and clinical abortions, increase the clinical pregnancy rate, and reduce the risks for the children born. These approaches may be simply the selection of embryos, since it has been shown that a rate of more than 50% fragmentations might be associated with a higher rate of chromosomal abnormalities and therefore with a higher rate of malformations in children born (Ebner et al. 2001). In this study malformation rates were 3.2%, 6.3%, 13.3%, and 36.4% after transfer of embryos with no fragments, with fewer than 25% fragments, with 25 to 50% fragments, and with more than 50% fragments, respectively (Ebner et al. 2001). Other risk factors, however, may be associated with "infertility" but might not be identified in the future. This is an important fact that couples have to be counselled about.

One problem, however, has been emphasized in nearly every chapter of this book concerning the influences on the different aspects of outcome of pregnancies and children born after ART. This problem is the high rate of multiple births – and, different from the problem "infertility-linked risk", is a problem that can be easily influenced!

Especially in IVF cycles, there have been many studies favouring even single embryo transfer in couples with a very high chance of conceiving (Vilska et al. 1999; Templeton 2000; Dhont 2001; Martikainen et al. 2001). Others have clearly shown that the strategy of elective two-embryo transfer in the UK does not lead to lower pregnancy rates in good-prognosis patients, but leads only to an increased risk of multiple pregnancies (Templeton and Morris 1998; Ozturk and Templeton 2002). Going straight to singleton pregnancies will lead to a substantial reduction in the risk of early and late pregnancy loss, in the number of pregnancy complications, the risk of premature birth and, therefore, the severe morbidity and mortality of the neonates.

Finally, the development of children after birth as well as the structures of ART families are not worse as compared to those created in a natural way. This is opposite to the critical view of different authors in the past and present literature. This is even true of families created with the help of a gamete donor – either oocyte donation or sperm donation. It is also true for a new kind of family, that headed by lesbian couples. It is more the quality of the relationship between the parents, of whatever gender, and the quality of care for the children, than that the family is of the traditional type, that makes a "good family".

Future studies, with a prospective and controlled design, should help to provide more knowledge on all these aspects of pregnancies and birth following any ART procedure. The data so far show that any new technique must be evaluated – in particular every cohort of infertile patients must be evaluated concerning the pattern of risks linked to that particular type of infertility.

One infertile patient is not the same infertile patient as another – not only with regard to the chosen and most successful treatment procedure, but also and perhaps more importantly with regard to the established pregnancy and subsequent health of the child born.

Abbreviation List

AC	amniocentesis
AFP	α fetoprotein
AID	assisted insemination with donor sperms
AIH	assisted insemination with husbands sperms
ART	assisted reproductive technologies
CI	confidence interval
CVS	chorionic villous sampling
ELSI	elongated spermatid injection
ESHRE	European Society of Human Reproduction and Embryology
ET	embryo transfer
FISH	fluorescent in situ hybridization
GIFT	gamete intrafallopian transfer
GnRH	gonadotropin releasing hormone
hCG	human chorionic gonadotropin
HMG	human menopausal gonadotropin
ICSI	intracytoplasmic sperm injection
IUI	intrauterine insemination
IVF	in vitro fertilization
MESA	microsurgical sperm aspiration
MOM	multiples of median
PCO	polycystic ovary syndrome
PIH	pregnancy-induced hypertension
PND	prenatal diagnosis
PROM	premature rupture of membranes
ROSI	round spermatid injection
SGA	small for gestational age
SUZI	subzonal insemination
TESE	testicular sperm extraction
USD	US dollars
ZIFT	zygote intrafallopian transfer

References

Abdalla HI, Billett A, Kan AK, Baig S, Wren M, Korea L, Studd JW (1998) Obstetric outcome in 232 ovum donation pregnancies. Br J Obstet Gynaecol 105:332–337

Abidin RR (1995) Parenting stress index: professional manual, 3rd edn. Psychological Assessment Resources, Odessa, FL

Aboulghar H, Aboulghar M, Mansour R, Serour G, Amin Y, Al-Inany H (2001) A prospective controlled study of karyotyping for 430 consecutive babies conceived through intracytoplasmic sperm injection. Fertil Steril 76:249–253

Achenbach TM (1991a) Manual for the child behavior checklist. University of Vermont, Department of Psychiatry, Burlington

Achenbach TM (1991b) Manual for the teachers' report form and 1991 profile. University of Vermont, Department of Psychiatry, Burlington

Adonakis G, Camus M, Joris H, Vandervorst M, Van Steirteghem A, Devroey P (1997) The role of the number of replaced embryos on intracytoplasmic sperm injection outcome in women over the age of 40. Hum Reprod 12:2542–2545

Ahuja KK, Mostyn BJ, Simons EG (1997) Egg sharing and egg donation: attitudes of British egg donors and recipients. Hum Reprod 12:2845–2852

Ahuja KK, Simons EG, Mostyn BJ, Bowen-Simpkins P (1998) An assessment of the motives and morals of egg share donors: policy of 'payments' to egg donors requires a fair review. Hum Reprod 13:2671–2678

Al Hasani S, Ludwig M, Gagsteiger F, Kupker W, Sturm R, Yilmaz A, Bauer O, Diedrich K (1996) Comparison of cryopreservation of supernumerary pronuclear human oocytes obtained after intracytoplasmic sperm injection (ICSI) and after conventional in-vitro fertilization. Hum Reprod 11:604–607

Al Hasani S, Ludwig M, Palermo I, Kupker W, Sandmann J, Johannisson R, Fornara P, Sturm R, Bals-Pratsch M, Bauer O, Diedrich K (1999) Intracytoplasmic injection of round and elongated spermatids from azoospermic patients: results and review. Hum Reprod 14 [Suppl 1]:97–107

Amuzu B, Laxova R, Shapiro SS (1990) Pregnancy outcome, health of children, and family adjustment after donor insemination. Obstet Gynecol 75:899–905

Antinori S, Versaci C, Gholami GH, Panci C, Caffa B (1993) Oocyte donation in menopausal women. Hum Reprod 8:1487–1490

Antoni K, Hamori M (2001) Distribution of fetal malformations and chromosomal disorders in 1290 ICSI newborns between 1993 and 2000. Hum Reprod (abstract book) 16:39

Applegarth L, Goldberg NC, Cholst I, McGoff N, Fantini D, Zellers N, Black A, Rosenwaks Z (1995) Families created through ovum donation: a preliminary investigation of obstetrical outcome and psychosocial adjustment. J Assist Reprod Genet 12:574–580

Asch RH, Vazquez ME, Verez JR, Stern JJ, Cerrillo M, Yerena C, Diaz L, Gutierrez NA (1999) Decreased frequency of chromosomal abnormalities in spontaneous abortions from in-vitro fertilization pregnancies: a prospective, controlled, ongoing study. Hum Reprod (abstract book) 14:100

Australian in vitro fertilisation collaborative group (1985) High incidence of preterm births and early losses in pregnancy after in vitro fertilisation. BMJ 291:1160–1163

Aytoz A, De Catte L, Camus M, Bonduelle M, Van Assche E, Liebaers I, Van Steirteghem A, Devroey P (1998) Obstetric outcome after prenatal diagnosis in pregnancies obtained after intracytoplasmic sperm injection. Hum Reprod 13:2958–2961

Aytoz A, Van den AE, Bonduelle M, Camus M, Joris H, Van Steirteghem A, Devroey P (1999) Obstetric outcome of pregnancies after the transfer of cryopreserved and fresh embryos obtained by conventional in-vitro fertilization and intracytoplasmic sperm injection. Hum Reprod 14:2619–2624

Baetens P, Devroey P, Camus M, Van Steirteghem AC, Ponjaert-Kristoffersen I (2000) Counselling couples and donors for oocyte donation: the decision to use either known or anonymous oocytes. Hum Reprod 15:476–484

Bajirova M, Francannet C, Pouly JL, de Mouzon J, Janny L (2001) FIVNAT Final report on the malformation risk after ICSI using epididymal or testicular spermatozoids. Hum Reprod (abstract book) 16:40

Baranov VS (1983) Effect of monosomy of the autosomes on the preimplantation stages of embryogenesis in laboratory mice. Ontogenez 14:73–81

Barkai G, Goldman B, Ries L, Chaki R, Dor J, Cuckle H (1996) Down's syndrome screening marker levels following assisted reproduction. Prenat Diagn 16:1111–1114

Barlow P, Lejeune B, Puissant F, Englert Y, Van Rysselberge M, Degueldre M, Vekemans M, Leroy F (1988) Early pregnancy loss and obstetrical risk after in-vitro fertilization and embryo replacement. Hum Reprod 3:671–675

Barros A, Sousa M, Oliveira C, Silva J, Almeida V, Beires J (1997) Pregnancy and birth after intracytoplasmic sperm injection with totally immotile sperm recovered from the ejaculate. Fertil Steril 67:1091–1094

Bartels I, Schlosser M, Bartz UG, Pauer HU (1998) Paternal origin of trisomy 21 following intracytoplasmic sperm injection (ICSI). Hum Reprod 13:3345–3346

Beck A, Steer R (1987) The Beck depression inventory manual. Psychological Corporation, San Antonio, CA

Beck A, Herrero J, Stalf T, Mehnert C, Gips H, Lang U (2001) High pregnancy risk and poorer perinatal outcome after IVF. Hum Reprod (abstract book) 16:140

Bene E, Anthony J (1985) Manual for the family relations test. NFER-Nelson, Windsor, UK

Beral V, Doyle P, Tan SL, Mason BA, Campbell S (1990) Outcome of pregnancies resulting from assisted conception. Br Med Bull 46:753–768

Bergh T, Ericson A, Hillensjo T, Nygren KG, Wennerholm UB (1999) Deliveries and children born after in-vitro fertilisation in Sweden 1982–1995: a retrospective cohort study. Lancet 354:1579–1585

Bernasko J, Lynch L, Lapinski R, Berkowitz RL (1997) Twin pregnancies conceived by assisted reproductive techniques: maternal and neonatal outcomes. Obstet Gynecol 89:368–372

Bewley S, Wright JT (1991) Maternal death associated with ovum donation twin pregnancy. Hum Reprod 6:898–899

Biggers JD (1981) In vitro fertilization and embryo transfer in human beings. N Engl J Med 304:336–342

Blanchette H (1993) Obstetric performance of patients after oocyte donation. Am J Obstet Gynecol 168:1803–1807

Bofinger MK, Needham DF, Saldana LR, Sosnowski JP, Blough RI (1999) 45,X/46,X,r(Y) karyotype transmitted by father to son after intracytoplasmic sperm injection for oligospermia. A case report. J Reprod Med 44:645–648

Bonduelle M, Desmyttere S, Buysse A, Van Assche E, Schietecatte J, Devroey P, Van Steirteghem AC, Liebaers I (1994) Prospective follow-up study of 55 children born after subzonal insemination and intracytoplasmic sperm injection. Hum Reprod 9:1765–1769

Bonduelle M, Legein J, Derde MP, Buysse A, Schietecatte J, Wisanto A, Devroey P, Van Steirteghem A, Liebaers I (1995a) Comparative follow-up study of 130 children born after intracytoplasmic sperm injection and 130 children born after in-vitro fertilization. Hum Reprod 10:3327–3331

Bonduelle M, Legein J, Wilikens A (1995b) Follow up study of children born after intra-cytoplasmatic sperm injection. Hum Reprod 10:52–54

Bonduelle M, Legein J, Buysse A, Van Assche E, Wisanto A, Devroey P, Van Steirteghem AC, Liebaers I (1996a) Prospective follow-up study of 423 children born after intracyto-plasmic sperm injection. Hum Reprod 11:1558–1564

Bonduelle M, Wilikens A, Buysse A, Van Assche E, Wisanto A, Devroey P, Van Steirteghem AC, Liebaers I (1996b) Prospective follow-up study of 877 children born after intracyto-plasmic sperm injection (ICSI), with ejaculated epididymal and testicular spermatozoa and after replacement of cryopreserved embryos obtained after ICSI. Hum Reprod 11 [Suppl 4]:131–155

Bonduelle M, Aytoz A, Wilikens A, Buysse A, Van Assche E, Devroey P, Van Steirteghem A, Liebaers I (1998a) Prospective follow-up study of 1987 children born after intracyto-plasmic sperm injection (ICSI). In: Filicori M, Flamigni C (eds) Treatment of infertility: the new frontiers. Communications Media for Education, New Jersey, pp 445–461

Bonduelle M, Joris H, Hofmans K, Liebaers I, Van Steirteghem A (1998b) Mental develop-ment of 201 ICSI children at 2 years of age. Lancet 351:1553

Bonduelle M, Wilikens A, Buysse A, Van Assche E, Devroey P, Van Steirteghem AC, Liebaers I (1998c) A follow-up study of children born after intracytoplasmic sperm injection (ICSI) with epididymal and testicular spermatozoa and after replacement of cryopreserved embryos obtained after ICSI. Hum Reprod 13 [Suppl 1]:196–207

Bonduelle M, Camus M, De Vos A, Staessen C, Tournaye H, Van Assche E, Verheyen G, Devroey P, Liebaers I, Van Steirteghem A (1999) Seven years of intracytoplasmic sperm injection and follow-up of 1987 subsequent children. Hum Reprod 14 [Suppl 1]: 243–264

Bonduelle M, Liebaers I, Deketelaere V, Derde MP, Camus M, Devroey P, Van Steirteghem A (2002) Neonatal data on a cohort of 2889 infants born after ICSI (1991–1999) and of 2995 infants born after IVF (1983–1999). Hum Reprod 17:671–694

Borini A, Bafaro G, Violini F, Bianchi L, Casadio V, Flamigni C (1995) Pregnancies in post-menopausal women over 50 years old in an oocyte donation program. Fertil Steril 63: 258–261

Boue JG, Boue A (1973) Increased frequency of chromosomal anomalies in abortions after induced ovulation. Lancet 1:679–680

Boue JG, Boue A (1976) Chromosomal anomalies in early spontaneous abortion. (Their consequences on early embryogenesis and in vitro growth of embryonic cells). Curr Top Pathol 62:193–208

Boue J, Bou A, Lazar P (1975) Retrospective and prospective epidemiological studies of 1500 karyotyped spontaneous human abortions. Teratology 12:11–26

Bourgain C, Devroey P, Van Waesberghe L, Smitz J, Van Steirteghem AC (1990) Effects of natural progesterone on the morphology of the endometrium in patients with primary ovarian failure. Hum Reprod 5:537–543

Brandes JM, Scher A, Itzkovits J, Thaler I, Sarid M, Gershoni-Baruch R (1992) Growth and development of children conceived by in vitro fertilization. Pediatrics 90:424–429

Brewaeys A, Ponjaert I, Van Hall EV, Golombok S (1997) Donor insemination: child develop-ment and family functioning in lesbian mother families. Hum Reprod 12:1349–1359

Brown GW, Rutter ML (1966) The measurement of family activities and relationships: a methodological study. Hum Relat 19:241–263

Bui TH, Wramsby H (1996) Micromanipulative assisted fertilization – still clinical research. Hum Reprod 11:925–926

Buitendijk SE (1999) Children after in vitro fertilization. An overview of the literature. Int J Technol Assess Health Care 15:52–65

Butler D (1995) Spermatid injection fertilizes ethics debate. Nature 377:277

Cahill DJ (1998) Risks of GnRH agonist administration in early pregnancy. In: Filicori M, Flamigni C (eds) Ovulation induction. Update '98. Parthenon Publishing Group, New York, pp 97–106

Cameron IT, Rogers PA, Caro C, Harman J, Healy DL, Leeton JF (1989) Oocyte donation: a review. Br J Obstet Gynaecol 96:893–899

Cano F, Simon C, Remohi J, Pellicer A (1995) Effect of aging on the female reproductive system: evidence for a role of uterine senescence in the decline in female fecundity. Fertil Steril 64:584–589

Causio F, Fischetto R, Schonauer LM, Leonetti T (1999) Intracytoplasmic sperm injection in infertile patients with structural cytogenetic abnormalities. J Reprod Med 44:859–864

Cayan S, Conaghan J, Schriock ED, Ryan IP, Black LD, Turek PJ (2001) Birth after intracytoplasmic sperm injection with use of testicular sperm from men with Kartagener/immotile cilia syndrome. Fertil Steril 76:612–614

Cederblad M, Höök B (1991) Östgötastudien-Stressreaktioner Och Beteendestörningar Hos Barn Pa 08-Talet i Östergötland

Cederblad M, Friberg B, Ploman F, Sjoberg NO, Stjernqvist K, Zackrisson E (1996) Intelligence and behaviour in children born after in-vitro fertilization treatment. Hum Reprod 11:2052–2057

Chan RW, Raboy B, Patterson CJ (1998) Psychosocial adjustment among children conceived via donor insemination by lesbian and heterosexual mothers. Child Dev 69:443–457

Chandley AC, Edmond P, Christie S, Gowans L, Fletcher J, Frackiewicz A, Newton M (1975) Cytogenetics and infertility in man. I. Karyotype and seminal analysis: results of a five-year survey of men attending a subfertility clinic. Ann Hum Genet 39:231–254

Chillon M, Casals T, Mercier B, Bassas L, Lissens W, Silber S, Romey MC, Ruiz-Romero J, Verlingue C, Claustres M (1995) Mutations in the cystic fibrosis gene in patients with congenital absence of the vas deferens. N Engl J Med 332:1475–1480

Chong AP, Taymor ML (1975) Sixteen years' experience with therapeutic donor insemination. Fertil Steril 26:791–795

Clayton CE, Kovacs GT (1982) AID offspring: initial follow-up study of 50 couples. Med J Aust 1:338–339

Cohen J, Mayaux MJ, Guihard-Moscato ML, Schwartz D (1986) In-vitro fertilization and embryo transfer: a collaborative study of 1163 pregnancies on the incidence and risk factors of ectopic pregnancies. Hum Reprod 1:255–258

Cohen J, Mayaux MJ, Guihard-Moscato ML (1988) Pregnancy outcomes after in vitro fertilization. A collaborative study on 2342 pregnancies. Ann NY Acad Sci 541:1–6

Cook R, Golombok S, Bish A, Murray C (1995) Disclosure of donor insemination: parental attitudes. Am J Orthopsychiatry 65:549–559

Cook R, Bradley S, Golombok S (1998) A preliminary study of parental stress and child behaviour in families with twins conceived by in-vitro fertilization. Hum Reprod 13:3244–3246

Cornet D, Alvarez S, Antoine JM, Tibi C, Mandelbaum J, Plachot M, Salat-Baroux J (1990) Pregnancies following ovum donation in gonadal dysgenesis. Hum Reprod 5:291–293

Couillin P, Ravise N, Afoutou JM, Chaibi R, Azoulay M, Hors J, Oury JF, Boue J, Boue A (1987) HLA and molar pregnancies (triploidies, hydatidiform moles and choriocarcinoma). Etiological and epidemiological study. Ann Genet 30:197–208

Coulam CB, Opsahl MS, Sherins RJ, Thorsell LP, Dorfmann A, Krysa L, Fugger E, Schulman JD (1996) Comparisons of pregnancy loss patterns after intracytoplasmic sperm injection and other assisted reproductive technologies. Fertil Steril 65:1157–1162

Craft I, Brinsden P (1989) Alternatives to IVF: the outcome of 1071 first GIFT procedures. Hum Reprod 4:29–36

Cranley MS (1981) Development of a tool for the measurement of maternal attachment during pregnancy. Nurs Res 30:281–284

Crawford BS, Davis J, Harrigill K (1997) Uterine artery atherosclerotic disease: histologic features and clinical correlation. Obstet Gynecol 90:210–215

Cruger D, Toft B, Agerholm I, Fedder J, Hald F, Bruun-Petersen G (2001) Birth of a healthy girl after ICSI with ejaculated spermatozoa from a man with non-mosaic Klinefelter's syndrome. Hum Reprod 16:1909–1911

Cummins JM, Jequier AM (1994) Treating male infertility needs more clinical andrology, not less. Hum Reprod 9:1214–1219

Daniels KR (1994) Adoption and donor insemination: factors influencing couples' choices. Child Welfare 73:5–14

David G, Czyglik F, Mayaux MJ, Martin-Boyce A, Schwartz D (1980) Artificial insemination with frozen sperm: protocol, method of analysis and results for 1188 women. Br J Obstet Gynaecol 87:1022–1028

De Catte L, Liebaers I, Foulon W, Bonduelle M, Van Assche E (1996) First trimester chorionic villus sampling in twin gestations. Am J Perinatol 13:413–417

de Mouzon J, Lancaster PA (1993) World collaborative report 1993. 15th world congress on fertility and sterility, Montepellier, France

de Ziegler D, Bessis R, Frydman R (1991) Vascular resistance of uterine arteries: physiological effects of estradiol and progesterone. Fertil Steril 55:775–779

Deutsches IVF Register (2000) DIR – Deutsches IVF Register 1999

Devroey P, Pados G (1998) Preparation of endometrium for egg donation. Hum Reprod Update 4:856–861

Devroey P, Smitz J, Camus M, Wisanto A, Deschacht J, Van Waesberghe L, Van Steirteghem AC (1989) Synchronization of donor's and recipient's cycles with GnRH analogues in an oocyte donation programme. Hum Reprod 4:270–274

Dhont M (2001) Single-embryo transfer. Semin Reprod Med 19:251–258

Dhont M, De Sutter P, Ruyssinck G, Martens G, Bekaert A (1999) Perinatal outcome of pregnancies after assisted reproduction: a case-control study. Am J Obstet Gynecol 181:688–695

D'Hooghe T, Debrock S, Rijkers A, Legius E, De Zegher F, Meuleman C, Vanderschueren D, Spitz B (2000) Is the prevalence of congenital abnormalities after ICSI increased? The Leuven data 1994–1999. Hum Reprod (abstract book) 15:128–129

Doyle P, Beral V, Maconochie N (1992) Preterm delivery, low birthweight and small-for-gestational-age in liveborn singleton babies resulting from in-vitro fertilization. Hum Reprod 7:425–428

D'Souza SW, Rivlin E, Cadman J, Richards B, Buck P, Lieberman BA (1997) Children conceived by in vitro fertilisation after fresh embryo transfer. Arch Dis Child Fetal Neonatal Ed 76:F70–F74

Ebner T, Yaman C, Moser M, Sommergruber M, Polz W, Tews G (2001) Embryo fragmentation in vitro and its impact on treatment and pregnancy outcome. Fertil Steril 76:281–285

Edwards RG (1992) Why are agonadal and post-amenorrhoeic women so fertile after oocyte donation? Hum Reprod 7:733–734

Egozcue S, Blanco J, Vendrell JM, Garcia F, Veiga A, Aran B, Barri PN, Vidal F, Egozcue J (2000) Human male infertility: chromosome anomalies, meiotic disorders, abnormal spermatozoa and recurrent abortion. Hum Reprod Update 6:93–105

Engel W, Murphy D, Schmid M (1996) Are there genetic risks associated with microassisted reproduction? Hum Reprod 11:2359–2370

Englert Y, Govaerts I (1998) Oocyte donation: particular technical and ethical aspects. Hum Reprod 13 [Suppl 2]:90–97

Englert Y, Rodesch C, Van den Bergh M, Bertrand E (1996) Oocyte shortage for donation may be overcome in a programme with anonymous permutation of related donors. Hum Reprod 11:2425–2428

Ericson A, Kallen B (2001) Congenital malformations in infants born after IVF: a population-based study. Hum Reprod 16:504–509

Ericson A, Nygren KG, Olausson PO, Kallen B (2002) Hospital care utilization of infants born after IVF. Hum Reprod 17:929–932

Evans MI, Hume RFJ, Polak S, Yaron Y, Drugan A, Diamond MP, Johnson MP (1997) The geriatric gravida: multifetal pregnancy reduction, donor eggs, and aggressive infertility treatments. Am J Obstet Gynecol 177:875–878

Fasouliotis SJ, Schenker JG (1996) Cryopreservation of embryos: medical, ethical, and legal issues. J Assist Reprod Genet 13:756–761

Fedorcsak P, Storeng R, Dale PO, Tanbo T, Abyholm T (2000) Obesity is a risk factor for early pregnancy loss after IVF or ICSI. Acta Obstet Gynecol Scand 79:43–48

Feichtinger W, Obruca A, Brunner M (1995) Sex chromosomal abnormalities and intracytoplasmic sperm injection. Lancet 346:1566

Ferguson-Smith MA (1983) Prenatal chromosome analysis and its impact on the birth incidence of chromosome disorders. Br Med Bull 39:355–364

Ferraris S, Silengo M, Ponzone A, Perugini L (1999) Goldenhar anomaly in one of triplets derived from in vitro fertilization. Am J Med Genet 84:167–168

Fielding D, Handley S, Duqueno L (1998) Motivation, attitudes and experience of donation: a follow-up of women donating eggs in assisted conception treatment. J Comm Appl Soc Psychol 8:273–287

Finkelhor D, Russell D (1984) Women as perpetrators: review of the evidence. In: Finkelhor D (ed) Child sexual abuse. Free Press, New York, pp 171–187

Foresta C, Ferlin A (2001) Offspring conceived by intracytoplasmic sperm injection. Lancet 358:1270

Fortuny A, Carrio A, Soler A, Cararach J, Fuster J, Salami C (1988) Detection of balanced chromosome rearrangements in 445 couples with repeated abortion and cytogenetic prenatal testing in carriers. Fertil Steril 49:774–779

Friedler S, Mordel N, Lipitz S, Mashiach S, Glezerman M, Laufer N (1994) Perinatal outcome of triplet pregnancies following assisted reproduction. J Assist Reprod Genet 11: 459–462

Friedman F Jr, Copperman AB, Brodman ML, Shah D, Sandler B, Grunfeld L (1996) Perinatal outcome after embryo transfer in ovum recipients. A comparison with standard in vitro fertilization. J Reprod Med 41:640–644

Frydman R, Belaisch-Allart J, Fries N, Hazout A, Glissant A, Testart J (1986) An obstetric assessment of the first 100 births from the in vitro fertilization program at Clamart, France. Am J Obstet Gynecol 154:550–555

Frydman R, Forman RG, Belaisch-Allart J, Hazout A, Fernandez H, Testart J (1989) An obstetric analysis of fifty consecutive pregnancies after transfer of cryopreserved human embryos. Am J Obstet Gynecol 160:209–213

Garel M, Blondel B (1992) Assessment at 1 year of the psychological consequences of having triplets. Hum Reprod 7:729–732

Garel M, Salobir C, Lelong N, Blondel B (2001) Development and behaviour of seven-year-old triplets. Acta Paediatr 90:539–543

Geipel A, Gembruch U, Ludwig M, Germer U, Schwinger E, Dormeier A, Diedrich K (1999) Genetic sonography as the preferred option of prenatal diagnosis in patients with pregnancies following intracytoplasmic sperm injection. Hum Reprod 14:2629–2634

German EK, Mukherjee T, Osborne D, Copperman AB (2001) Does increasing ovum donor compensation lead to differences in donor characteristics? Fertil Steril JID 76:75–79

Gleicher N, Campbell DP, Chan CL, Karande V, Rao R, Balin M, Pratt D (1995) The desire for multiple births in couples with infertility problems contradicts present practice patterns. Hum Reprod 10:1079–1084

Goldfarb J, Kinzer DJ, Boyle M, Kurit D (1996) Attitudes of in vitro fertilization and intrauterine insemination couples toward multiple gestation pregnancy and multifetal pregnancy reduction. Fertil Steril 65:815–820

Golombok S, Cook R, Bish A, Murray C (1993) Quality of parenting in families created by the new reproductive technologies: a brief report of preliminary findings. J Psychosom Obstet Gynaecol 14 [Suppl]:17–22

Golombok S, Brewaeys A, Cook R, Giavazzi MT, Guerra D, Mantovani A, van Hall E, Crosignani PG, Dexeus S (1996) The European study of assisted reproduction families: family functioning and child development. Hum Reprod 11:2324–2331

Golombok S, Murray C, Brinsden P, Abdalla H (1999) Social versus biological parenting: family functioning and the socioemotional development of children conceived by egg or sperm donation. J Child Psychol Psychiatry 40:519–527

Golombok S, Spencer A, Rutter M (1983) Children in lesbian and single-parent households: psychosexual and psychiatric appraisal. J Child Psychol Psychiatry 24:551–572

Gosden RG (1973) Chromosomal anomalies of preimplantation mouse embryos in relation to maternal age. J Reprod Fertil 35:351–354

Gottlieb C, Lalos O, Lindblad F (2000) Disclosure of donor insemination to the child: the impact of Swedish legislation on couples' attitudes. Hum Reprod 15:2052–2056

Gottman JS (1990) Homosexuality and family relations. In: Bozett FW, Sussman MB (eds) Children of gay and lesbian parents. Harrington Park, New York, pp 177–196

Govaerts I, Englert Y, Vamos E, Rodesch F (1995) Sex chromosome abnormalities after intracytoplasmic sperm injection. Lancet 346:1095–1096

Govaerts I, Koenig I, Van den BM, Bertrand E, Revelard P, Englert Y (1996) Is intracytoplasmic sperm injection (ICSI) a safe procedure? What do we learn from early pregnancy data about ICSI? Hum Reprod 11:440–443

Govaerts I, Devreker F, Koenig I, Place I, Van den Bergh M, Englert Y (1998) Comparison of pregnancy outcome after intracytoplasmic sperm injection and in-vitro fertilization. Hum Reprod 13:1514–1518

Green R (1974) Sexual identity conflict in children and adults. Basic Books, New York

Green R (1978) Sexual identity of 37 children raised by homosexual or transsexual parents. Am J Psychiatry 135:692–697

Green R, Mandel JB, Hotvedt ME, Gray J, Smith L (1986) Lesbian mothers and their children: a comparison with solo parent heterosexual mothers and their children. Arch Sex Behav 15:167–184

Grefenstette I, Royere D, Barthelemy C, Tharanne MJ, Lansac J (1990) Outcome of 470 pregnancies after artificial insemination with frozen sperm. J Gynecol Obstet Biol Reprod (Paris) 19:737–744

Griffith R (1970) The abilities of young children. Child development research centre, London

Hansen M, Kurinczuk JJ, Bower C, Webb S (2002) The risk of major birth defects after intracytoplasmic sperm injection and in vitro fertilization. N Engl J Med 346:725–730

Hanson FW, Tennant FR, Zorn EM, Samuels S (1985) Analysis of 2136 genetic amniocenteses: experience of a single physician. Am J Obstet Gynecol 152:436–443

Harris J, Kallen B, Robert E (1995) Descriptive epidemiology of alimentary tract atresia. Teratology 52:15–29

Harris MB, Turner PH (1985) Gay and lesbian parents. J Homosex 12:101–113

Harter S, Pike R (1984) The pictorial scale of perceived competence and social acceptance for young children. Child Dev 55:1969–1982

Heijnsbroek I, Helmerhorst FM, van den Berg-Helder AF, van der Zwan KJ, Naaktgeboren N, Keirse MJ (1995) Follow-up of 30 pregnancies after embryo cryopreservation. Eur J Obstet Gynecol Reprod Biol 59:201–204

Hennebicq S, Pelletier R, Bergues U, Rousseaux S (2001) Risk of trisomy 21 in offspring of patients with Klinefelter's syndrome. Lancet 357:2104–2105

Hens L, Bonduelle M, Liebaers I, Devroey P, Van Steirteghem AC (1988) Chromosome aberrations in 500 couples referred for in-vitro fertilization or related fertility treatment. Hum Reprod 3:451–457

Hewitson L, Martinovich C, Takahashi D, Schatten G (2000) Elongated spermatid injection (ELSI) in the rhesus monkey. Fertil Steril 74 [Suppl 1]:S67

Hirsch P, Wurfel W, Fiedler K, Krusmann G, Rothenaicher M (1989) Amniotic fluid puncture for prenatal diagnosis in IVF pregnancy – 1985–1987 results. Gynakol Rundsch 29 [Suppl 2]:441–443

Ho ML, Chen JY, Ling UP, Chen JH, Huang CM, Chang CC, Su PH (1996) Changing epidemiology of triplet pregnancy: etiology and outcome over twelve years. Am J Perinatol 13:269–275

Hoeffer B (1981) Children's acquisition of sex-role behavior in lesbian-mother families. Am J Orthopsychiatry 51:536–544

Hong SJ, Choi BC, Song JH, Paik EC, Koong MK, Jun JH, Kim JW, Jun JY, Kang IS (1999) Frequency of chromosomal abnormalities in spontaneous abortions from in-vitro fertilization pregnancy: does assisted reproduction treatment affect incidence of chromosomal abnormalities. Hum Reprod (abstract book) 14:60

Hook EB (1981) Rates of chromosome abnormalities at different maternal ages. Obstet Gynecol 58:282–285

Horne G, Jamaludin A, Critchlow JD, Falconer DA, Newman MC, Oghoetuoma J, Pease EH, Lieberman BA (1998) A 3 year retrospective review of intrauterine insemination, using cryopreserved donor spermatozoa and cycle monitoring by urinary or serum luteinizing hormone measurements. Hum Reprod 13:3045–3048

Hsiung CH, Karow WG, Gentry WC, Tsui M, Smith DW, Tejada RI (1987) The first reported case of Down syndrome in the Southern California Fertility Institute's in vitro fertilization and embryo transfer program. J In Vitro Fertil Embryo Transf 4:312–315

Huggins SL (1989) A comparative study of self-esteem of adolescent children of divorced lesbian mothers and divorced heterosexual mothers. Harrington Park, New York

Hulvert J, Mardesic T, Voboril J, Muller P (1999) Heterotopic pregnancy and its occurrence in assisted reproduction. Ceska Gynekol 64:299–301

In't Velt P, Brandenburg H, Verhoeff A, Dhont M, Los F (1995a) Sex chromosomal abnormalities and intracytoplasmic sperm injection. Lancet 346:773

In't Velt P, van Opstal D, Van den Berg C, Van Ooijen M, Brandenburg H, Pijpers L, Jahoda MG, Stijnen TH, Los FJ (1995b) Increased incidence of cytogenetic abnormalities in chorionic villus samples from pregnancies established by in vitro fertilization and embryo transfer (IVF-ET). Prenat Diagn 15:975–980

Jacobs PA, Browne C, Gregson N, Joyce C, White H (1992) Estimates of the frequency of chromosome abnormalities detectable in unselected newborns using moderate levels of banding. J Med Genet 29:103–108

Jahoda MG, Brandenburg H, Reuss A, Cohen-Overbeek TE, Wladimiroff JW, Los FJ, Sachs ES (1991) Transcervical (TC) and transabdominal (TA) CVS for prenatal diagnosis in Rotterdam: experience with 3611 cases. Prenat Diagn 11:559–561

Jones BM, MacFarlane K (eds) (1980) Sexual abuse of children: selected readings. Free Press, New York

Jones HW Jr, Acosta AA, Andrews MC, Garcia JE, Jones GS, Mantzavinos T, McDowell J, Sandow BA, Veeck L, Whibley TW (1983) What is a pregnancy? A question for programs of in vitro fertilization. Fertil Steril 40:728–733

Kalfoglou AL, Gittelsohn J (2000) A qualitative follow-up study of women's experiences with oocyte donation. Hum Reprod 15:798–805

Kallen B, Castilla EE, Kringelbach M, Lancaster PA, Martinez-Frias ML, Mastroiacovo P, Mutchinick O, Robert E (1991) Parental fertility and infant hypospadias: an international case-control study. Teratology 44:629–634

Kallen B, Martinez-Frias ML, Castilla EE (1992) Hormone therapy during pregnancy and isolated hypospadias: an international case-control study. Int J Risk Safety Med 3:182–188

Kanyo K, Konc J (2000) A follow-up study of children born after non-contact laser-assisted hatching at 96 deliveries, 134 babies. Hum Reprod (abstract book) 15:63

Katzorke T, Propping D, Tauber PF (1981) Results of donor artificial insemination (AID) in 415 couples. Int J Fertil 26:260–266

Khamsi F, Endman MW, Lacanna IC, Wong J (1997) Some psychological aspects of oocyte donation from known donors on altruistic basis. Fertil Steril 68:323–327

Kirkpatrick M (1987) Clinical implications of lesbian mother studies. J Homosex 14:201–211

Kirkpatrick M, Smith C, Roy R (1981) Lesbian mothers and their children: a comparative survey. Am J Orthopsychiatry 51:545–551

Klyman CM (1986) Pregnancy as a reaction to early childhood sibling loss. J Am Acad Psychoanal 14:323–335

Kohlberg L (1964) Development of moral character and moral ideology. In: Hoffman ML, Hoffman LW (eds) Review of child development research. Russell Sage, New York, pp 383–431

Koudstaal J, Braat DD, Bruinse HW, Naaktgeboren N, Vermeiden JP, Visser GH (2000a) Obstetric outcome of singleton pregnancies after IVF: a matched control study in four Dutch university hospitals. Hum Reprod 15:1819–1825

Koudstaal J, Bruinse HW, Helmerhorst FM, Vermeiden JP, Willemsen WN, Visser GH (2000b) Obstetric outcome of twin pregnancies after in-vitro fertilization: a matched control study in four Dutch university hospitals. Hum Reprod 15:935–940

Koulischer L, Verloes A, Lesenfants S, Jamar M, Herens C (1997) Genetic risk in natural and medically assisted procreation. Early Pregnancy 3:164–171

Kurinczuk JJ, Bower C (1997) Birth defects in infants conceived by intracytoplasmic sperm injection: an alternative interpretation. BMJ 315:1260–1265

Lahat E, Raziel A, Friedler S, Schieber-Kazir M, Ron-El R (1999) Long-term follow-up of children born after inadvertent administration of a gonadotrophin-releasing hormone agonist in early pregnancy. Hum Reprod 14:2656–2660

Laing SC, Gosden RG, Fraser HM (1984) Cytogenetic analysis of mouse oocytes after experimental induction of follicular overripening. J Reprod Fertil 70:387–393

Lambalk CB, van Hooff M (2001) Natural versus induced twinning and pregnancy outcome: a Dutch nationwide survey of primiparous dizygotic twin deliveries. Fertil Steril 75:731–736

Lancaster PA (1985) Obstetric outcome. Clin Obstet Gynaecol 12:847–864

Lancaster PA (1986) Health registers for congenital malformations and in vitro fertilization. Clin Reprod Fertil 4:27–37

Lancaster PA (1987) Congenital malformations after in-vitro fertilisation. Lancet 2:1392–1393

Lancaster PA (1989) High incidence of selected congenital malformations after assisted conception. Teratology 40:288

Lancaster PA (1996) Registers of in-vitro fertilization and assisted conception. Hum Reprod 11 [Suppl 4]:89–104

Lancaster PA, Hust T, Shafir E (2000) Congenital malformations and other pregnancy outcome after microinsemination. Reprod Toxicol 14:74

Lansac J, Imbault M, Lecomte C, Magnin G, Moxhon E, Tharanne MJ, Berger C (1983) Pregnancy and labor after insemination with frozen sperm from a donor. J Gynecol Obstet Biol Reprod (Paris) 12:511–518

Lansac J, Thepot F, Mayaux MJ, Czyglick F, Wack T, Selva J, Jalbert P (1997) Pregnancy outcome after artificial insemination or IVF with frozen semen donor: a collaborative study of the French CECOS Federation on 21,597 pregnancies. Eur J Obstet Gynecol Reprod Biol 74:223–228

Lass A, Croucher C, Duffy S, Dawson K, Margara R, Winston RM (1998) One thousand initiated cycles of in vitro fertilization in women or = 40 years of age. Fertil Steril 70:1030–1034

le Porrier N, Thepot F, Cmier B, Herlicoviez M, Herlicoviez D, Obry E, Sauvalle A, Alliet J (1988) Etude cytogenetique des produits de fausses couches precoces apres fecondation in vitro. Contracept Fertil Sex 16:652–653

Legro RS, Wong IL, Paulson RJ, Lobo RA, Sauer MV (1995) Recipient's age does not adversely affect pregnancy outcome after oocyte donation. Am J Obstet Gynecol 172:96–100

Levran D, Ben Shlomo I, Dor J, Ben Rafael Z, Nebel L, Mashiach S (1991) Aging of endometrium and oocytes: observations on conception and abortion rates in an egg donation model. Fertil Steril 56:1091–1094

Liebaers I, Bonduelle M, Van Assche E, Devroey P, Van Steirteghem A (1995) Sex chromosome abnormalities after intracytoplasmic sperm injection. Lancet 346:1095

Lindenberg S, Lauritsen JG, Lenz S (1985) Ectopic pregnancy and spontaneous abortions following in-vitro fertilization and embryo transfer. Acta Obstet Gynecol Scand 64:31–34

Locke HJ, Wallace KM (1959) Short marital-adjustment and predictions tests: their reliability and validity. Marr Fam Living 21:251–255

Loft A, Petersen K, Erb K, Mikkelsen AL, Grinsted J, Hald F, Hindkjaer J, Nielsen KM, Lundstrom P, Gabrielsen A, Lenz S, Hornnes P, Ziebe S, Ejdrup HB, Lindhard A, Zhou Y, Nyboe AA (1999) A Danish national cohort of 730 infants born after intracytoplasmic sperm injection (ICSI) 1994–1997. Hum Reprod 14:2143–2148

Ludwig M, Al-Hasani S, Ghasemi M, Gizycki U, Küpker W, Diedrich K (1999a) Intrazytoplasmatische Spermatozoeninjektion – ICSI (II): Geburt und Gesundheit von 267 Kindern. Geburtsh Frauenheilkd 59:399

Ludwig M, Geipel A, Küpker W, Al-Hasani S, Ghasemi M, Gizycki U, Diedrich K (1999b) Intrazytoplasmatische Spermieninjektion – ICSI (I): Verlauf von 310 Schwangerschaften und Ergebnisse der Pränataldiagnostik. Geburtsh Frauenheilkd 59:387–394

Ludwig M, Riethmuller-Winzen H, Felberbaum RE, Olivennes F, Albano C, Devroey P, Diedrich K (2001a) Health of 227 children born after controlled ovarian stimulation for in vitro fertilization using the luteinizing hormone-releasing hormone antagonist cetrorelix. Fertil Steril 75:18–22

Ludwig M, Schröder AK, Diedrich K (2001b) Impact of intracytoplasmic sperm injection on the activation and fertilization process of oocytes. RBMonline 3:228–238

Lutjen P, Trounson A, Leeton J, Findlay J, Wood C, Renou P (1984) The establishment and maintenance of pregnancy using in vitro fertilization and embryo donation in a patient with primary ovarian failure. Nature 307:174–175

Ma S, Robinson W, Lam R, Yuen BH (2001) Maternal origin of monosomy 21 derived from ICSI. Hum Reprod 16:1100–1103

Machin GA, Crolla JA (1974) Chromosome constitution of 500 infants dying during the perinatal period. With an appendix concerning other genetic disorders among these infants. Humangenetik 23:183–198

Macnab AJ, Zouves C (1991) Hypospadias after assisted reproduction incorporating in vitro fertilization and gamete intrafallopian transfer. Fertil Steril 56:918–922

Maman E, Lunenfeld E, Levy A, Vardi H, Potashnik G (1998) Obstetric outcome of singleton pregnancies conceived by in vitro fertilization and ovulation induction compared with those conceived spontaneously. Fertil Steril 70:240–245

Mantzavinos T, Kanakas N, Zourlas PA (1996) Heterotopic pregnancies in an in-vitro fertilization program. Clin Exp Obstet Gynecol 23:205–208

Marcus SF, Brinsden PR (1995) Analysis of the incidence and risk factors associated with ectopic pregnancy following in-vitro fertilization and embryo transfer. Hum Reprod 10:199–203

Marcus SF, Macnamee M, Brinsden P (1995) The prediction of ectopic pregnancy after in-vitro fertilization and embryo transfer. Hum Reprod 10:2165–2168

Marino B, Marcelletti C (1989) Complex congenital heart disease after in vitro fertilization. Am J Dis Child 143:1136–1137

Maroulis GB (1991) Effect of aging on fertility and pregnancy. Semin Reprod Endocrinol 9:165–175

Martikainen H, Tiitinen A, Tomas C, Tapanainen J, Orava M, Tuomivaara L, Vilska S, Hyden-Granskog C, Hovatta O (2001) One versus two embryo transfer after IVF and ICSI: a randomized study. Hum Reprod 16:1900–1903

Martin RH (1984) Comparison of chromosomal abnormalities in hamster egg and human sperm pronuclei. Biol Reprod 31:819–825

Martin RH (1996) The risk of chromosomal abnormalities following ICSI. Hum Reprod 11:924–925

Mau G (1981) Progestins during pregnancy and hypospadias. Teratology 24:285–287

Maudlin I, Fraser LR (1977) The effect of PMSG dose on the incidence of chromosomal anomalies in mouse embryos fertilized in vitro. J Reprod Fertil 50:275–280

Maudlin I, Fraser LR (1978) Maternal age and the incidence of aneuploidy in first-cleavage mouse embryos. J Reprod Fertil 54:423–426

Maymon R, Shulman A (2001) Comparison of triple serum screening and pregnancy outcome in oocyte donation versus IVF pregnancies. Hum Reprod 16:691–695

Maymon R, Dreazen E, Tovbin Y, Bukovsky I, Weinraub Z, Herman A (1999) The feasibility of nuchal translucency measurement in higher order multiple gestations achieved by assisted reproduction. Hum Reprod 14:2102–2105

Meirow D, Schenker JG (1995) Appraisal of gamete intrafallopian transfer. Eur J Obstet Gynecol Reprod Biol 58:59–65

Meschede D, Horst J (1997) Sex chromosomal anomalies in pregnancies conceived through intracytoplasmic sperm injection: a case for genetic counselling. Hum Reprod 12: 1125–1127

Meschede D, Lemcke B, Exeler JR, De Geyter C, Behre HM, Nieschlag E, Horst J (1998a) Chromosome abnormalities in 447 couples undergoing intracytoplasmic sperm injection-prevalence, types, sex distribution and reproductive relevance. Hum Reprod 13: 576–582

Meschede D, Lemcke B, Stussel J, Louwen F, Horst J (1998b) Strong preference for non-invasive prenatal diagnosis in women pregnant through intracytoplasmic sperm injection (ICSI). Prenat Diagn 18:700–705

Meschede D, Lemcke B, Behre HM, Geyter CD, Nieschlag E, Horst J (2000) Non-reproductive heritable disorders in infertile couples and their first degree relatives. Hum Reprod 15: 1609–1612

Mesrogli M, Nitsche U, Maas DH, Degenhardt F, Dieterle S, Schlosser HW (1991) Rate of early abortion after in vitro fertilization and embryo transfer. Geburtshilfe Frauenheilkd 51:688–693

Michalas S, Loutradis D, Drakakis P, Milingos S, Papageorgiou J, Kallianidis K, Koumantakis E, Aravantinos D (1996) Oocyte donation to women over 40 years of age: pregnancy complications. Eur J Obstet Gynecol Reprod Biol 64:175–178

Miller JF, Williamson E, Glue J, Gordon YB, Grudzinskas JG, Sykes A (1980) Fetal loss after implantation. A prospective study. Lancet 2:554–556

Monni G, Cau G, Lai R, Demontis G, Usai V (1999) Intracytoplasmic sperm injection and prenatal invasive diagnosis. Prenat Diagn 19:390

Moomjy M, Mangieri R, Beltramone F, Cholst I, Veeck L, Rosenwaks Z (2000) Shared oocyte donation: society's benefits. Fertil Steril 73:1165–1169

Morin NC, Wirth FH, Johnson DH, Frank LM, Presburg HJ, Van der Water VL, Chee EM, Mills JL (1989) Congenital malformations and psychosocial development in children conceived by in vitro fertilization. J Pediatr 115:222–227

Munne S, Lee A, Rosenwaks Z, Grifo J, Cohen J (1993) Diagnosis of major chromosome aneuploidies in human preimplantation embryos. Hum Reprod 8:2185–2191

Munne S, Alikani M, Tomkin G, Grifo J, Cohen J (1995) Embryo morphology, developmental rates, and maternal age are correlated with chromosome abnormalities. Fertil Steril 64:382–391

Murray C, Golombok S (2000) Oocyte and semen donation: a survey of UK licensed centres. Hum Reprod 15:2133–2139

Mushin DN, Barreda-Hanson MC, Spensley JC (1986) In vitro fertilization children: early psychosocial development. J In Vitro Fertil Embryo Transf 3:247–252

Neveux LM, Palomaki GE, Knight GJ, Haddow JE (1996) Multiple marker screening for Down syndrome in twin pregnancies. Prenat Diagn 16:29–34

New Zealand Government (1977) Human rights commission act. Government Printer, Wellington

New Zealand Government (1987) Status of children amendment act. Government Printer, Wellington

New Zealand Government (1993) Human rights act. Government Printer, Wellington

Nielsen J (1975) Chromosome examination of newborn children: purpose and ethical aspects. Humangenetik 26:215–222

Nielsen J, Wohlert M (1991) Chromosome abnormalities found among 34,910 newborn children: results from a 13-year incidence study in Arhus, Denmark. Hum Genet 87:81–83

No authors listed (2000) Assisted reproductive technology in the United States: 1997 results generated from the American Society for Reproductive Medicine/Society for Assisted Reproductive Technology Registry. Fertil Steril 74:641–653, discussion 653–654

Noyes RW, Nertig A, Rock J (1950) Dating the endometrial biopsy. Fertil Steril 1:3–25

Ogura A, Yanagimachi R (1995) Spermatids as male gametes. Reprod Fertil Dev 7:155–158

Olivennes F, Schneider Z, Remy V, Blanchet V, Kerbrat V, Fanchin R, Hazout A, Glissant M, Fernandez H, Dehan M, Frydman R (1996) Perinatal outcome and follow-up of 82 children aged 1–9 years old conceived from cryopreserved embryos. Hum Reprod 11: 1565–1568

Ozturk O, Templeton A (2002) In-vitro fertilisation and risk of multiple pregnancy. Lancet 359:232

Pados G, Camus M, Van Waesberghe L, Liebaers I, Van Steirteghem A, Devroey P (1992) Oocyte and embryo donation: evaluation of 412 consecutive trials. Hum Reprod 7: 1111–1117

Pados G, Camus M, Van Steirteghem A, Bonduelle M, Devroey P (1994) The evolution and outcome of pregnancies from oocyte donation. Hum Reprod 9:538–542

Page DC, Silber S, Brown LG (1999) Men with infertility caused by AZFc deletion can produce sons by intracytoplasmic sperm injection, but are likely to transmit the deletion and infertility. Hum Reprod 14:1722–1726

Palermo G, Joris H, Devroey P, Van Steirteghem AC (1992) Pregnancies after intracytoplasmic injection of single spermatozoon into an oocyte. Lancet 340:17–18

Palermo GD, Colombero LT, Schattman GL, Davis OK, Rosenwaks Z (1996) Evolution of pregnancies and initial follow-up of newborns delivered after intracytoplasmic sperm injection. JAMA 276:1893–1897

Papaligoura Z, Panopoulou-Maratou O, Solman M, Arvaniti K (2001) Development of infants conceived after intracytoplasmic sperm injection. Hum Reprod (abstract book) 16:83

Patrat C, Wolf JP, Epelboin S, Hugues JN, Olivennes F, Granet P, Zorn JR, Jouannet P (1999) Pregnancies, growth and development of children conceived by subzonal injection of spermatozoa. Hum Reprod 14:2404–2410

Paulson RJ, Hatch IE, Lobo RA, Sauer MV (1997a) Cumulative conception and live birth rates after oocyte donation: implications regarding endometrial receptivity. Hum Reprod 12:835–839

Paulson RJ, Thornton MH, Francis MM, Salvador HS (1997b) Successful pregnancy in a 63-year-old woman. Fertil Steril 67:949–951

Pellestor F, Sele B (1988) Assessment of aneuploidy in the human female by using cytogenetics of IVF failures. Am J Hum Genet 42:274–283

Pergament E, Schulman JD, Copeland K, Fine B, Black SH, Ginsberg NA, Frederiksen MC, Carpenter RJ (1992) The risk and efficacy of chorionic villus sampling in multiple gestations. Prenat Diagn 12:377–384

Perrot-Applanat M, Groyer-Picard MT, Garcia E, Lorenzo F, Milgrom E (1988) Immunocytochemical demonstration of estrogen and progesterone receptors in muscle cells of uterine arteries in rabbits and humans. Endocrinology 123:1511–1519

Persson JW, Peters GB, Saunders DM (1996) Is ICSI associated with risks of genetic disease? Implications for counselling, practice and research. Hum Reprod 11:921–924

Peschka B, Leygraaf J, Van der Ven K, Montag M, Schartmann B, Schubert R, van der Ven H, Schwanitz G (1999) Type and frequency of chromosome aberrations in 781 couples undergoing intracytoplasmic sperm injection. Hum Reprod 14:2257–2263

Petersen K, Hornnes PJ, Ellingsen S, Jensen F, Brocks V, Starup J, Jacobsen JR, Andersen AN (1995) Perinatal outcome after in vitro fertilisation. Acta Obstet Gynecol Scand 74:129–131

Pezeshki K, Feldman J, Stein DE, Lobel SM, Grazi RV (2000) Bleeding and spontaneous abortion after therapy for infertility. Fertil Steril JID 74:504–508

Place I, Englert Y (2001) A prospective longitudinal study of singleton ICSI children compared to IVF and spontaneously conceived children shows no difference in psychomotor and intellectual development over the whole preschool period. Hum Reprod (abstract book) 16:83

Plachot M (1989) Chromosome analysis of spontaneous abortions after IVF. A European survey. Hum Reprod 4:425–429

Plachot M (1997) The human oocyte. Genetic aspects. Ann Genet 40:115–120

Plachot M, de Grouchy J, Junca AM, Mandelbaum J, Salat-Baroux J, Cohen J (1988a) Chromosome analysis of human oocytes and embryos: does delayed fertilization increase chromosome imbalance? Hum Reprod 3:125–127

Plachot M, de Grouchy J, Junca AM, Mandelbaum J, Turleau C, Couillin P, Cohen J, Salat-Baroux J (1987a) From oocyte to embryo: a model, deduced from in vitro fertilization, for natural selection against chromosome abnormalities. Ann Genet 30:22–32

Plachot M, Junca AM, Mandelbaum J, de Grouchy J, Salat-Baroux J, Cohen J (1986) Chromosome investigations in early life. I. Human oocytes recovered in an IVF programme. Hum Reprod 1:547–551

Plachot M, Junca AM, Mandelbaum J, de Grouchy J, Salat-Baroux J, Cohen J (1987b) Chromosome investigations in early life. II. Human preimplantation embryos. Hum Reprod 2:29–35

Plachot M, Veiga A, Montagut J, de Grouchy J, Calderon G, Lepretre S, Junca AM, Santalo J, Carles E, Mandelbaum J (1988b) Are clinical and biological IVF parameters correlated with chromosomal disorders in early life: a multicentric study. Hum Reprod 3:627–635

Porcu E, Dal Prato L, Seracchioli R, Petracchi S, Fabbri R, Flamigni C (1997) Births after transcervical gamete intrafallopian transfer with a falloposcopic delivery system. Fertil Steril 67:1175–1177

Puryear D (1983) A comparison between the children of lesbian mothers and the children of heterosexual mothers. Unpublished doctoral dissertation. California School of Professional Psychology, Berkeley, CA

Quinton D, Rutter M (1988) Parenting breakdown: the making and breaking of intergenerational links. Avebury Gower Publishing, Aldershot, UK

Quinton D, Rutter M, Rowlands O (1976) An evaluation of an interview assessment of marriage. Psychol Med 6:577–586

Raoul-Duval A, Letur-Konirsch H, Frydman R (1992) Anonymous oocyte donation: a psychological study of recipients, donors and children. Hum Reprod 7:51–54

Raoul-Duval A, Bertrand-Servais M, Letur-Konirsch H, Frydman R (1994) Psychological follow-up of children born after in-vitro fertilization. Hum Reprod 9:1097–1101

Rappaport VJ, Dominguez CE, Hunt KS (1998) Genetic abnormalities and effects on reproduction. Infert Reprod Med Clin North Am 9:607–633

Raziel A, Friedler S, Herman A, Strassburger D, Maymon R, Ron-El R (1997) Recurrent heterotopic pregnancy after repeated in-vitro fertilization treatment. Hum Reprod 12:1810–1812

Rees RL (1979) A comparison of children of lesbian and single heterosexual mothers on three measurements of socialisation. Unpublished doctoral dissertation. California School of Professional Psychology, Berkeley, CA

Reijo R, Alagappan RK, Patrizio P, Page DC (1996) Severe oligozoospermia resulting from deletions of azoospermia factor gene on Y chromosome. Lancet 347:1290–1293

Retief AE, Van Zyl JA, Menkveld R, Fox MF, Kotze GM, Brusnicky J (1984) Chromosome studies in 496 infertile males with a sperm count below 10 million/ml. Hum Genet 66: 162–164

Reubinoff BE, Samueloff A, Ben-Haim M, Friedler S, Schenker JG, Lewin A (1997) Is the obstetric outcome of in vitro fertilized singleton gestations different from natural ones? A controlled study. Fertil Steril 67:1077–1083

Ribbert LS, Kornman LH, De Wolf BT, Simons AH, Jansen CA, Beekhuis JR, Mantingh A (1996) Maternal serum screening for fetal Down syndrome in IVF pregnancies. Prenat Diagn 16:35–38

Rizk B, Doyle P, Tan SL, Rainsbury P, Betts J, Brinsden P, Edwards R (1991a) Perinatal outcome and congenital malformations in in-vitro fertilization babies from the Bourn-
Hallam group. Hum Reprod 6:1259–1264

Rizk B, Tan SL, Morcos S, Riddle A, Brinsden P, Mason BA, Edwards RG (1991b) Heterotopic
pregnancies after in vitro fertilization and embryo transfer. Am. J Obstet Gynecol
164:161–164

Roesler M, Wise L, Katayama KP (1989) Karyotype analysis of blighted ova in pregnancies
achieved by in vitro fertilization. Fertil Steril 51:1065–1066

Rogers PA, Leeton J, Cameron IT, Murphy C, Healy DL, Lutjen P (1988) Oocyte donation. In:
Wood E, Trounson A (eds) Clinical in-vitro fertilization. Berlin, Springer, Berlin Heidelberg New York, pp 143–154

Ron-El R, Lahat E, Golan A, Lerman M, Bukovsky I, Herman A (1994) Development of
children born after ovarian superovulation induced by long-acting gonadotropin-
releasing hormone agonist and menotropins, and by in vitro fertilization. J Pediatr
125:734–737

Rosenberg H, Epstein Y (1995) Follow-up study of anonymous ovum donors. Hum Reprod
10:2741–2747

Rosenwaks Z (1987) Donor eggs: their application in modern reproductive technologies.
Fertil Steril 47:895–909

Ruble DN, Brooks-Gunn J, Fleming AS, Fitzmaurice G, Stangor C, Deutsch F (1990) Transi-
tion to motherhood and the self: measurement, stability, and change. J Pers Soc Psychol
58:450–463

Rufat P, Olivennes F, de Mouzon J, Dehan M, Frydman R (1994) Task force report on the
outcome of pregnancies and children conceived by in vitro fertilization (France: 1987 to
1989). Fertil Steril 61:324–330

Rust J, Bennun I, Crowe M, Golombok S (1988) The handbook of the Golombok rust
inventory of marital state. NFER-Nelson, Windsor, UK

Rutter M, Tizard J, Whitmore K (1970) Education, health and behavior. Longman, London,
UK

Santalo J, Badenas J, Catala V, Egozcue J (1987) Chromosomes of mouse embryos in vivo
and in vitro: effect of manipulation, maternal age and gamete ageing. Hum Reprod
2:717–719

Sarafino EP (1979) An estimate of nationwide incidence of sexual offences against children.
Child Welfare 58:127–134

SART (1992) In vitro fertilization-embryo transfer (IVF-ET) in the United States: 1990
results from the IVF-ET Registry. Medical Research International. Society for Assisted
Reproductive Technology (SART), The American Fertility Society. Fertil Steril 57:
15–24

SART (2002) Assisted reproductive technology in the United States: 1998 results generated
from the American Society for Reproductive Medicine/Society for Assisted Reproductive
Technology Registry. Fertil Steril 77:18–31

Sauer MV, Paulson RJ (1992) Oocyte donors: a demographic analysis of women at the
University of Southern California. Hum Reprod 7:726–728

Sauer MV, Paulson RJ, Lobo RA (1990) A preliminary report on oocyte donation extending
reproductive potential to women over 40. N Engl J Med 323:1157–1160

Sauer MV, Paulson RJ, Lobo RA (1992) Reversing the natural decline in human fertility.
An extended clinical trial of oocyte donation to women of advanced reproductive age.
JAMA 268:1275–1279

Sauer MV, Miles RA, Dahmoush L, Paulson RJ, Press M, Moyer D (1993) Evaluating the effect
of age on endometrial responsiveness to hormone replacement therapy: a histologic
ultrasonographic, and tissue receptor analysis. J Assist Reprod Genet 10:47–52

Sauer MV, Paulson RJ, Lobo RA (1995) Pregnancy in women 50 or more years of age:
outcomes of 22 consecutively established pregnancies from oocyte donation. Fertil
Steril 64:111–115

Sauer MV, Paulson RJ, Lobo RA (1996) Oocyte donation to women of advanced reproductive age: pregnancy results and obstetrical outcomes in patients 45 years and older. Hum Reprod 11:2540–2543

Saunders DM, Mathews M, Lancaster PA (1988) The Australian Register: current research and future role. A preliminary report. Ann NY Acad Sci 541:7–21

Saunders K, Spensley J, Munro J, Halasz G (1996) Growth and physical outcome of children conceived by in vitro fertilization. Pediatrics 97:688–692

Sbracia M, Baldi M, Cao D, Sandrelli A, Chiandetti A, Poverini R, Aragona C (2002) Preferential location of sex chromosomes, their aneuploidy in human sperm, and their role in determining sex chromosome aneuploidy in embryos after ICSI. Hum Reprod 17: 320–324

Schattman GL, Rosenwaks Z, Berkely A (1995) Congenital malformations in children born utilizing the assisted reproductive technologies 36. Serono international symposium on genetics of gametes and embryos, 2–5 June, New York

Schieve LA, Meikle SF, Ferre C, Peterson HB, Jeng G, Wilcox LS (2002) Low and very low birth weight in infants conceived with use of assisted reproductive technology. N Engl J Med 346:731–737

Schlesselman JJ (1979) How does one assess the risk of abnormalities from human in vitro fertilization? Am J Obstet Gynecol 135:135–148

Schmidt-Sarosi C, Schwartz LB, Lublin J, Kaplan-Grazi D, Sarosi P, Perle MA (1998) Chromosomal analysis of early fetal losses in relation to transvaginal ultrasonographic detection of fetal heart motion after infertility. Fertil Steril 69:274–277

Scholtes MC, Behrend C, Dietzel-Dahmen J, van Hoogstraten DG, Marx K, Wohlers S, Verhoeven H, Zeilmaker GH (1998) Chromosomal aberrations in couples undergoing intracytoplasmic sperm injection: influence on implantation and ongoing pregnancy rates. Fertil Steril 70:933–937

Schover LR, Collins RL, Quigley MM, Blankstein J, Kanoti G (1991) Psychological follow-up of women evaluated as oocyte donors. Hum Reprod 6:1487–1491

Schover LR, Rothmann SA, Collins RL (1992) The personality and motivation of semen donors: a comparison with oocyte donors. Hum Reprod 7:575–579

Schover LR, Thomas AJ, Falcone T, Attaran M, Goldberg J (1998) Attitudes about genetic risk of couples undergoing in-vitro fertilization. Hum Reprod 13:862–866

Schröder AK, Diedrich K, Ludwig M (2001) Fertilization and preimplantation development after intracytoplasmic sperm injection. 3:247

Schwartz D, Mayaux MJ, Guihard-Moscato ML, Czyglik F, David G (1986) Abortion rate in A.I.D. and semen characteristics: a study of 1345 pregnancies. Andrologia 18:292–298

Sengoku K, Dukelow RW (1988) Gonadotropin effects on chromosomal normality of hamster preimplantation embryos. Biol Reprod 38:150–155

Seppala M (1985) The world collaborative report on in vitro fertilization and embryo replacement: current state of the art in January 1984. Ann NY Acad Sci 442:558–563

Serhal P (1990) Oocyte donation and surrogacy. Br Med Bull 46:796–812

Serour GI, Aboulghar M, Mansour R, Sattar MA, Amin Y, Aboulghar H (1998) Complications of medically assisted conception in 3,500 cycles. Fertil Steril 70:638–642

Shenfield F, Steele SJ (1997) What are the effects of anonymity and secrecy on the welfare of the child in gamete donation? Hum Reprod 12:392–395

Shields LE, Serafini PC, Schenken RS, Moore CM (1992) Chromosomal analysis of pregnancy losses in patients undergoing assisted reproduction. J Assist Reprod Genet 9:57–60

Shozu M, Akimoto K, Tanaka J, Sonoda Y, Inoue M, Michikura Y (1997) Antenatal detection of Meckel-Gruber syndrome in only one dizygotic twin following in vitro fertilization and embryo transfer. Gynecol Obstet Invest 43:142–144

Silver RI, Rodriguez R, Chang TS, Gearhart JP (1999) In vitro fertilization is associated with an increased risk of hypospadias. J Urol 161:1954–1957

Simon A, Holzer H, Hurwitz A, Revel A, Zentner BS, Lossos F, Laufer N (1998) Comparison of cryopreservation outcome following intracytoplasmic sperm injection and conventional in vitro fertilization. J Assist Reprod Genet 15:431–437

Simpson JL (1980) Genes, chromosomes, and reproductive failure. Fertil Steril 33:107–116

Snijders RJ, Johnson S, Sebire NJ, Noble PL, Nicolaides KH (1996) First-trimester ultrasound screening for chromosomal defects. Ultrasound Obstet Gynecol 7:216–226

Snow MH (1975) Embryonic development of tetraploid mice during the second half of gestation. J Embryol Exp Morphol 34:707–721

Soderstrom-Anttila V, Sajaniemi N, Tiitinen A, Hovatta O (1998) Health and development of children born after oocyte donation compared with that of those born after in-vitro fertilization, and parents' attitudes regarding secrecy. Hum Reprod 13:2009–2015

Sonntag B, Meschede D, Ullmann V, Gassner P, Horst J, Nieschlag E, Behre HM (2001) Low-level sex chromosome mosaicism in female partners of couples undergoing ICSI therapy does not significantly affect treatment outcome. Hum Reprod 16:1648–1652

Spielberger C (1983) The handbook of the state-trait anxiety inventory. Consulting Psychologists Press, Palo Alto, CA

Spielmann H, Kruger C, Stauber M, Vogel R (1985) Abnormal chromosome behavior in human oocytes which remained unfertilized during human in vitro fertilization. J In Vitro Fertil Embryo Transf 2:138–142

Steptoe PC, Edwards RG (1976) Reimplantation of a human embryo with subsequent tubal pregnancy. Lancet 1:880–882

Stern JJ, Dorfmann AD, Gutierrez-Najar AJ, Cerrillo M, Coulam CB (1996) Frequency of abnormal karyotypes among abortuses from women with and without a history of recurrent spontaneous abortion. Fertil Steril 65:250–253

Strain L, Dean JC, Hamilton MP, Bonthron DT (1998) A true hermaphrodite chimera resulting from embryo amalgamation after in vitro fertilization. N Engl J Med 338: 166–169

Strandell A, Thorburn J, Hamberger L (1999) Risk factors for ectopic pregnancy in assisted reproduction. Fertil Steril 71:282–286

Strömberg B, Dahlquist G, Ericson A, Finnström O, Köster M, Stjernqvist K (2002) Neurological sequelae in children born after in-vitro fertilisation: a population based study. Lancet 359:461–465

Sunde A, Von D, V, Kahn JA, Molne K (1990) IVF in the Nordic countries 1981–1987: a collaborative survey. Hum Reprod 5:959–964

Sundstrom P, Wramsby H (1989) Evaluation of variations in pregnancy rates, implantation rates and early abortion rates within an in-vitro fertilization programme. Hum Reprod 4:443–445

Sutcliffe AG, D'Souza SW, Cadman J, Richards B, McKinlay IA, Lieberman B (1995a) Minor congenital anomalies, major congenital malformations and development in children conceived from cryopreserved embryos. Hum Reprod 10:3332–3337

Sutcliffe AG, D'Souza SW, Cadman J, Richards B, McKinlay IA, Lieberman B (1995b) Outcome in children from cryopreserved embryos. Arch Dis Child 72:290–293

Sutcliffe AG, Taylor B, Li J, Thornton S, Grudzinskas JG, Lieberman BA (1999) Children born after intracytoplasmic sperm injection: population control study. BMJ 318:704–705

Sutcliffe AG, Taylor B, Saunders K, Thornton S, Lieberman BA, Grudzinskas JG (2001) Outcome in the second year of life after in-vitro fertilisation by intracytoplasmic sperm injection: a UK case-control study. Lancet 357:2080–2084

Svare J, Norup P, Grove TS, Hornnes P, Maigaard S, Helm P, Petersen K, Nyboe AA (1993) Heterotopic pregnancies after in-vitro fertilization and embryo transfer – a Danish survey. Hum Reprod 8:116–118

Sweet RA, Schrott HG, Kurland R, Culp OS (1974) Study of the incidence of hypospadias in Rochester, Minnesota, 1940–1970, and a case-control comparison of possible etiologic factors. Mayo Clin Proc 49:52–58

Tabor A, Philip J, Madsen M, Bang J, Obel EB, Norgaard-Pedersen B (1986) Randomised controlled trial of genetic amniocentesis in 4606 low-risk women. Lancet 1:1287–93

Takagi N, Sasaki M (1976) Digynic triploidy after superovulation in mice. Nature 264:278–281

Tallo CP, Vohr B, Oh W, Rubin LP, Seifer DB, Haning RVJ (1995) Maternal and neonatal morbidity associated with in vitro fertilization. J Pediatr 127:794–800

Tan SL, Riddle A, Sharma A (1989) The relation between the number of gestational sacs seen after in-vitro fertilization and embryo transfer and outcome of pregnancy. Proceedings of the XIIth Asian and Oceanic Congress of Obstetrics and Gynecology

Tan SL, Doyle P, Campbell S, Beral V, Rizk B, Brinsden P, Mason B, Edwards RG (1992) Obstetric outcome of in vitro fertilization pregnancies compared with normally conceived pregnancies. Am J Obstet Gynecol 167:778–784

Tarlatzis BC (1996) Report on the activities of the ESHRE Task Force on intracytoplasmic sperm injection. European Society of Human Reproduction and Embryology. Hum Reprod 11 [Suppl 4]:160–185

Tarlatzis BC, Bili H (1998) Survey on intracytoplasmic sperm injection: report from the ESHRE ICSI Task Force. European Society of Human Reproduction and Embryology. Hum Reprod 13 [Suppl 1]:165–177

Tarlatzis BC, Bili H (2000) Intracytoplasmic sperm injection. Survey of world results. Ann NY Acad Sci 900:336–344

Tasker F, Golombok S (1995) Adults raised as children in lesbian families. Am J Orthopsychiatry 65:203–215

Tejada MI, Mendoza R, Carbonero K, Lizarraga MA, Escudero F, Benito JA (1990) Deletion of chromosome 4: 46,XY, del(4) (q31.3) after gamete intrafallopian transfer and in vitro fertilization-embryo transfer. Fertil Steril 54:953–954

Templeton A (2000) Avoiding multiple pregnancies in ART: replace as many embryos as you like-one at a time. Hum Reprod 15:1662

Templeton A, Morris JK (1998) Reducing the risk of multiple births by transfer of two embryos after in vitro fertilization. N Engl J Med 339:573–577

Testart J, Plachot M, Mandelbaum J, Salat-Baroux J, Frydman R, Cohen J (1992) World collaborative report on IVF-ET and GIFT: 1989 results. Hum Reprod 7:362–369

Testart J, Gautier E, Brami C, Rolet F, Sedbon E, Thebault A (1996) Intracytoplasmic sperm injection in infertile patients with structural chromosome abnormalities. Hum Reprod 11:2609–2612

Thepot F, Mayaux MJ, Czyglick F, Wack T, Selva J, Jalbert P (1996) Incidence of birth defects after artificial insemination with frozen donor spermatozoa: a collaborative study of the French CECOS Federation on 11,535 pregnancies. Hum Reprod 11:2319–2323

Trounson A, Leeton J, Besanko M, Wood C, Conti A (1983) Pregnancy established in an infertile patient after transfer of a donated embryo fertilised in vitro. Br Med J (Clin Res) 286:835–838

Tummon IS, Whitmore NA, Daniel SA, Nisker JA, Yuzpe AA (1994) Transferring more embryos increases risk of heterotopic pregnancy. Fertil Steril 61:1065–1067

Tunon K, Eik-Nes SH, Grottum P, Von D, V, Kahn JA (2000) Gestational age in pregnancies conceived after in vitro fertilization: a comparison between age assessed from oocyte retrieval, crown-rump length and biparietal diameter. Ultrasound Obstet Gynecol 15:41–46

Turner AJ, Coyle A (2000) What does it mean to be a donor offspring? The identity experiences of adults conceived by donor insemination and the implications for counselling and therapy. Hum Reprod 15:2041–2051

Urman B, Alatas C, Aksoy S, Mercan R, Nuhoglu A, Mumcu A, Isiklar A, Balaban B (2002) Transfer at the blastocyst stage of embryos derived from testicular round spermatid injection. Hum Reprod 17:741–743

Van Golde R, Boada M, Veiga A, Evers J, Geraedts J, Barri P (1999) A retrospective follow-up study on intracytoplasmic sperm injection. J Assist Reprod Genet 16:227–232

Van Opstal D, Los FJ, Ramlakhan S, Van Hemel JO, Van Den Ouweland AM, Brandenburg H, Pieters MH, Verhoeff A, Vermeer MC, Dhont M, In't VP (1997) Determination of the parent of origin in nine cases of prenatally detected chromosome aberrations found after intracytoplasmic sperm injection. Hum Reprod 12:682–686

Van Steirteghem A, Pados G, Devroey P, Bonduelle M, Van Assche E, Liebaers I (1992) Oocyte donation for genetic indications. Reprod Fertil Dev 4:681–688

Van Steirteghem AC, Van den Abbal E, Camus M, Van Waesberghe L, Braeckmans P, Khan I, Nijs M, Smitz J, Staessen C, Wisanto A (1987) Cryopreservation of human embryos obtained after gamete intra-Fallopian transfer and/or in-vitro fertilization. Hum Reprod 2:593–598

Van Steirteghem AC, Nagy Z, Joris H, Liu J, Staessen C, Smitz J, Wisanto A, Devroey P (1993) High fertilization and implantation rates after intracytoplasmic sperm injection. Hum Reprod 8:1061–1066

Van Steirteghem AC, Van der Elst J, Van den Abbal E, Joris H, Camus M, Devroey P (1994) Cryopreservation of supernumerary multicellular human embryos obtained after intra-cytoplasmic sperm injection. Fertil Steril 62:775–780

Varma TR, Patel RH (1987) Outcome of pregnancy following investigation and treatment of infertility. Int J Gynaecol Obstet 25:113–120

Vilska S, Tiitinen A, Hyden-Granskog C, Hovatta O (1999) Elective transfer of one embryo results in an acceptable pregnancy rate and eliminates the risk of multiple birth. Hum Reprod 14:2392–2395

Virro MR, Shewchuk AB (1984) Pregnancy outcome in 242 conceptions after artificial insemination with donor sperm and effects of maternal age on the prognosis for successful pregnancy. Am. J Obstet Gynecol 148:518–524

Wada I, Macnamee MC, Wick K, Bradfield JM, Brinsden PR (1994) Birth characteristics and perinatal outcome of babies conceived from cryopreserved embryos. Hum Reprod 9:543–546

Wald NJ, White N, Morris JK, Huttly WJ, Canick JA (1999) Serum markers for Down's syndrome in women who have had in vitro fertilisation: implications for antenatal screening. Br J Obstet Gynaecol 106:1304–1306

Wapner RJ, Johnson A, Davis G, Urban A, Morgan P, Jackson L (1993) Prenatal diagnosis in twin gestations: a comparison between second-trimester amniocentesis and first-trimester chorionic villus sampling. Obstet Gynecol 82:49–56

Weil E, Cornet D, Sibony C, Mandelbaum J, Salat-Baroux J (1994) Psychological aspects in anonymous and non-anonymous oocyte donation. Hum Reprod 9:1344–1347

Wennerholm UB, Bergh C (2000) Obstetric outcome and follow-up of children born after in vitro fertilization (IVF). Hum Fertil (Camb) 3:52–64

Wennerholm UB, Janson PO, Wennergren M, Kjellmer I (1991) Pregnancy complications and short-term follow-up of infants born after in vitro fertilization and embryo transfer (IVF/ET). Acta Obstet Gynecol Scand 70:565–573

Wennerholm UB, Bergh C, Hamberger L, Nilsson L, Reismer E, Wennergren M, Wikland M (1996) Obstetric and perinatal outcome of pregnancies following intracytoplasmic sperm injection. Hum Reprod 11:1113–1119

Wennerholm UB, Hamberger L, Nilsson L, Wennergren M, Wikland M, Bergh C (1997) Obstetric and perinatal outcome of children conceived from cryopreserved embryos. Hum Reprod 12:1819–1825

Wennerholm UB, Albertsson-Wikland K, Bergh C, Hamberger L, Niklasson A, Nilsson L, Thiringer K, Wennergren M, Wikland M, Borres MP (1998) Postnatal growth and health in children born after cryopreservation as embryos. Lancet 351:1085–1090

Wennerholm UB, Bergh C, Hamberger L, Lundin K, Nilsson L, Wikland M, Kallen B (2000a) Incidence of congenital malformations in children born after ICSI. Hum Reprod 15:944–948

Wennerholm UB, Bergh C, Hamberger L, Westlander G, Wikland M, Wood M (2000b) Obstetric outcome of pregnancies following ICSI, classified according to sperm origin and quality. Hum Reprod 15:1189–1194

Westergaard HB, Johansen AM, Erb K, Andersen AN (1999) Danish National In-Vitro Fertilization Registry 1994 and 1995: a controlled study of births, malformations and cytogenetic findings. Hum Reprod 14:1896–1902

Westergaard HB, Johansen AM, Erb K, Andersen AN (2000) Danish National IVF Registry 1994 and 1995. Treatment, pregnancy outcome and complications during pregnancy. Acta Obstet Gynecol Scand 79:384–389

Whitman-Elia GF, Plouffe LJ, Craft K, Khan I (1997) Esophageal atresia in an in vitro fertilization pregnancy. South Med J 90:86–88

Wilcox AJ, Weinberg CR, O'Connor JF, Baird DD, Schlatterer JP, Canfield RE, Armstrong EG, Nisula BC (1988) Incidence of early loss of pregnancy. N Engl J Med 319:189–194

Wimmers MS, van der Merwe JV (1988) Chromosome studies on early human embryos fertilized in vitro. Hum Reprod 3:894–900

Wisanto A, Magnus M, Bonduelle M, Liu J, Camus M, Tournaye H, Liebaers I, Van Steirteghem AC, Devroey P (1995) Obstetric outcome of 424 pregnancies after intracytoplasmic sperm injection. Hum Reprod 10:2713–2718

Wisanto A, Bonduelle M, Camus M, Tournaye H, Magnus M, Liebaers I, Van Steirteghem, A, Devroey P (1996) Obstetric outcome of 904 pregnancies after intracytoplasmic sperm injection. Hum Reprod [Suppl 4]:121–129

Wolff KM, McMahon MJ, Kuller JA, Walmer DK, Meyer WR (1997) Advanced maternal age and perinatal outcome: oocyte recipiency versus natural conception. Obstet Gynecol 89:519–523

Wood C, Trounson A (1985) Current state and future of IVF. Clin Obstet Gynaecol 12:753–766

Würfel W, Haas-Andela H, Krusmann G, Rothenaicher M, Hirsch P, Kwapisz HK, Haas J, Hogemann I, Fiedler K (1992) Prenatal diagnosis by amniocentesis in 82 pregnancies after in vitro fertilization. Eur J Obstet Gynecol Reprod Biol 44:47–52

Yanagimachi R (1995) Is an animal model needed for intracytoplasmic sperm injection (ICSI) and other assisted reproductive technologies? Hum Reprod 10:2525–2526

Yaron Y, Amit A, Brenner SM, Peyser MR, David MP, Lessing JB (1995) In vitro fertilization and oocyte donation in women 45 years of age and older. Fertil Steril 63:71–76

Yovich JL, Parry TS, French NP, Grauaug AA (1986) Developmental assessment of twenty in vitro fertilization (IVF) infants at their first birthday. J In Vitro Fertil Embryo Transf 3:253–257

Yovich JL, Mulcahy M, Matson P (1987) IVF and Goldenhar syndrome. J Med Genet 24:644

Zech H, Vanderzwalmen P, Prapas Y, Lejeune B, Duba E, Schoysman R (2000) Congenital malformations after intracytoplasmic injection of spermatids. Hum Reprod 15:969–971